To Jer

D0912112

FOOD, SEX & YOU

Best Wishes,

Stacey Gorlicky

FOOD, SEX & YOU

Untangling Body Obsession in a Weight-Obsessed World

STACEY GORLICKY

REGISTERED PSYCHOTHERAPIST

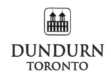

DUNDURN
TORONTO

Copy editor: Natalie Meditsky
Design: Jennifer Gallinger
Cover design: Sarah Beaudin
Cover image: Adapted from "Papaya series" by THOR.
Printer: Webcom

The Twelve Steps of Alcoholics Anonymous adapted with permission of Alcoholics Anonymous World Services, Inc. ("A.A.W.S.") Permission to adapt the Twelve Steps does not mean that A.A.W.S. has reviewed or approved the contents of this publication, or that A.A.W.S. necessarily agrees with the views expressed herein. A.A. is a program of recovery from alcoholism only — use of the Twelve Steps in connection with programs and activities which are patterned after A.A., but which address other problems, or in any other non-A.A. context, does not imply otherwise.

Library and Archives Canada Cataloguing in Publication

Gorlicky, Stacey, author
        Food, sex, and you : untangling body obsession in a
weight-obsessed world / Stacey Gorlicky.

Includes bibliographical references.
Issued in print and electronic formats.
ISBN 978-1-4597-3442-5 (paperback).--ISBN 978-1-4597-3443-2
(pdf).--ISBN 978-1-4597-3444-9 (epub)

        1. Self-acceptance. 2. Food--Psychological aspects.
3. Sex (Psychology). 4. Compulsive eaters. 5. Sex Addicts.
6. Addicts--Rehabilitation. I. Title.

BF575.S37G67 2016   158.1   C2015-908162-9
                                                      C2015-908163-7

1   2   3   4   5   20   19   18   17   16

 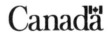 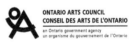

We acknowledge the support of the **Canada Council for the Arts** and the **Ontario Arts Council** for our publishing program. We also acknowledge the financial support of the **Government of Canada** through the **Canada Book Fund** and **Livres Canada Books**, and the **Government of Ontario** through the **Ontario Book Publishing Tax Credit** and the **Ontario Media Development Corporation**.

Care has been taken to trace the ownership of copyright material used in this book. The author and the publisher welcome any information enabling them to rectify any references or credits in subsequent editions.
— *J. Kirk Howard, President*

The publisher is not responsible for websites or their content unless they are owned by the publisher.

Printed and bound in Canada.

VISIT US AT
Dundurn.com | @dundurnpress | Facebook.com/dundurnpress | Pinterest.com/dundurnpress

Dundurn
3 Church Street, Suite 500
Toronto, Ontario, Canada
M5E 1M2

I dedicate this book to you, the reader.

I also dedicate this book to my family.
I am blessed to have so much love surrounding me.

CONTENTS

FOREWORD

BY LANCE LEVY, B.SC., M.B., CH.B., M.SC., FRCPC

Author of *Conquering Obesity: Deceptions in the Marketplace and the Real Story* and *Understanding Obesity: The Five Medical Causes*

I am honoured and delighted to have been asked to write the foreword to *Food, Sex, and You*. This is an excellent book on a topic very close to my research interests. As a consultant physician-scientist whose research is focused on discovering the reasons for treatment failures in adults who remain obese and food-addicted despite many diet interventions, I found this book sensitively written, accurate in detail, and full of excellent case histories from which my own patients take great comfort. Many details in the book are drawn from Stacey's own history of struggling with self-acceptance. She, too, had an unhealthy relationship with food, her body shape, and her weight, developed while living in an emotionally chaotic and weight- and size-obsessed world. Her understanding of how her childhood and teenage environment affected her self-concept and her eating was the key; it eventually allowed her to successfully carry out genuine changes in how she felt about herself and her world, and started her on a path toward healthy self-acceptance.

She has combined her understanding of the particular psychological issues frequently associated with the development of food addiction, binge eating, and obesity (chaotic family environment in childhood and adolescence; exposure to emotional, physical, or sexual abuse; alcoholic or drug-addicted parents or caregivers; and so forth) with the knowledge that genetically derived neurochemical imbalances (meaning imbalances that were present from early childhood and have genetic or epi-genetic roots) add to the difficulty of recovery because they can cause chronically poor sleep, an anxious or depressed mood, impulse control problems, and attentional problems, in addition to eating dis-regulation.

In most of the client cases she discusses, medication would be considered essential to support the beneficial effects of psychotherapy.

This book captures what medical science now knows about the origins and factors sustaining food addiction and obesity. The factors sustaining obesity, food addiction, and sex addiction are as follows:

1. Mood problems such as feelings of anxiety, pessimism, hopelessness, worthlessness, fatigue, poor self-esteem, and an inability to take enjoyment from pursuits that are usually pleasurable are some of the signals of a depressive mood that is of sufficient intensity to drain much of a person's energy. This makes attempts to successfully deal with addiction much less effective unless treatment of the mood is also undertaken, usually by combining medication with cognitive behavioural therapy and mindfulness-based stress reduction.

2. Chronic daytime fatigue is a symptom of many conditions. If the cause is not determined and corrected, food management, mood management, and weight control cannot be achieved.

3. Chronic pain is often a trigger for overuse of food, alcohol, and drugs, and can be diagnosed and treated much of the time.

4. Chronic stomach upset such as recurrent heartburn or acid reflux limits an individual's ability to correctly read the signals for hunger and fullness, and thus to respond correctly. It is easily diagnosed and when

treated successfully, makes food control much easier
to achieve.

5. Impulse regulation disorders — including binge-eating
    disorder and bulimia nervosa, nighttime eating syn-
    drome, and Attention Deficit Hyperactivity Disorder
    — are commonly missed. If undiagnosed, these disor-
    ders make control over eating behaviour, weight, sexual
    addiction, and sleep unmanageable by therapy alone.

There is much to be learned from Stacey's book, and I highly recommend it to the lay reader who may have some of the problems discussed. It
is obvious that binge eating, sex addiction, and ADHD are not character
flaws, but are instead true symptoms of medical problems, for which very
good treatments are available.

INTRODUCTION

The need for food and the desire for sex are two of the most power-ful engines driving evolution. Yet every day, as a psychotherapist, I am confronted with clients who fear one or both. Their sometimes bizarre stories might be hard for me to understand if I hadn't lived through many of the same nightmare scenarios myself.

By age nine, I believed that beauty was a woman's only passport to a happy, secure life. By age twelve, I was exercising a couple of hours every day, comparing myself to models in magazines, and wondering how to achieve their perfect figures. By age seventeen, I had a full-blown food addiction, which caused me to binge on ice cream, chocolate, and peanut butter, then purge with laxatives, exercise to total exhaustion, and restrict my diet to egg whites and water. Food — its indulgence and avoidance — was the focus of my life, and since I hated my out-of-control body, I feared and avoided sex.

In my decades of struggle, I tried every possible approach — mental, physical, emotional, spiritual — in my search for peace from my addiction. This included various therapies: Overeaters Anonymous, weekend work-shops, prescription drugs, private weight-loss clinics, inner-child work, dream interpretation, Sandplay, yoga, meditation, tantric sex, and so forth.

What worked? Nothing … and everything. Each new experience pre-pared me for the next level in discovering who I had been, who I was, and who I could become.

To replace the void left by my addiction, I knew I would need something BIG that I cared passionately about. Helping others transform their lives became my calling. I enrolled as a full-time student at Toronto's Transformational Arts College of Spiritual and Holistic Training, then followed up with other courses, including grief counselling, and then addiction counselling at McMaster University. This formal training provided me with methods and protocols to supplement what I had already learned, aided by wise mentors, through my own raw experience.

Though *Food, Sex, and You* addresses the vital connection between food and sex, it isn't just another guide to losing weight or how-to techniques to spice up a relationship. It's about helping you, as a reader, to recognize within yourself any obsession with, or fear of, these two powerful drives, and to embark on a voyage of self-discovery into the powerful childhood and cultural influences that have shaped you. In my experience, both personal and professional, obsessing over ten pounds can be as self-destructive as obsessing over sixty pounds. Both are addictions arising from a distorted body image, and are often cloaked in layers of denial.[1]

Women today — bombarded with Photoshopped images of supermodels and of our own pictures posted on Facebook and Tumblr — are becoming obsessed with their appearance at an earlier age than ever before.

Consider these statistics:

- In a 2008 Public Health Agency of Canada study, "In Healthy Settings for Young People in Canada," 37 percent of girls in grade nine and 40 percent in grade ten said they were too fat. Even among students of normal weight (based on body mass index, or BMI, the measure of body fat content based on a person's height and weight), 19 percent believed that they were too fat, and 12 percent reported trying to lose weight.
- In a 2002 Ministry of Health Canada survey, 1.5 percent of women aged fifteen to twenty-four admitted to suffering from an eating disorder.[2]

- According to a U.S. Youth Risk Behavior Survey, conducted between October 2004 and January 2006 by the U.S. Department of Health and Human Services, 61.7 percent of female students and 30 percent of male students were trying to lose weight.
- In 2000, the *Journal of the American Dietetic Association* published a study indicating that a significant number of five-year-old girls whose mothers dieted associated food restriction with thinness.
- According to the U.S. National Eating Disorders Association, 50 percent of adolescent girls will, at some point, have an eating disorder.

We have a crisis in our society when it comes to food and diet. One that shows no signs of going away.

Food, Sex, and You is for you if you feel uncomfortable about your body; if you fear you aren't "perfect" enough compared to women on TV and in magazines; if you obsess about your weight; if you hide your eating habits; if you turn to food for comfort; if you yo-yo diet; if you avoid mirrors; if you weigh yourself too often and beat yourself up when the "wrong" number pops up on the scale; if you binge then restrict; if you use laxatives, vomit, or over-exercise as a form of weight control; if you have been told by worried friends and relatives that you're too thin; if you are facing health issues related to obesity; or if you have been diagnosed with an eating disorder.

Food, Sex, and You is also for you if you avoid sex because you feel ashamed of your body; if you undress in the bathroom rather than in front of your partner or roommates; if you insist on having sex in the dark; if you hide your sexual self inside layers of fat; if you fear the predatory instincts of *all* men; if you believe that owning your sexuality may turn you into a "slut" in your own eyes or in the eyes of others; if you feel cheated of intimacy and sexual freedom because of alienation from your physical self. It's for anyone who fails to set safe emotional and physical boundaries in sexual relationships in an over-desire to please; who always chooses the wrong partners, or who has become addicted to sex to fill an inner vacuum.

It's for anyone who wants to break free from the shackles of self-judgment and dissatisfaction connected with either food or sex.

Food, Sex, and You is divided into three sections. In part one, "Addiction," I tell the story of my own eating disorder in unsparing detail — its severity, my fear of sex, and how it felt to hit rock bottom. In part two, "Recovery," I trace my journey through a minefield of possibilities, failures, and successes. An important first step was my joining Overeaters Anonymous. Just as critical was my discovery of the role that my undiagnosed ADHD (Attention Deficit Hyperactivity Disorder) played in my inability to control my bingeing. The weekend I spent learning about tantric sex launched me on another fantastic journey.

In part three, "Paying It Forward," I relate some of the touching stories told to me by my clients (whose names I have changed to protect identities), as both cautionary tales and sources of inspiration. Because addiction is addiction is addiction, I describe how drug abuse also feeds into eating and sexual disorders, and vice versa. Though the majority of my clients are women, I include stories of men's struggles with these issues, too. I also describe the treatment, both holistic and practical, that I offer my clients: how to compile a list of "danger" foods that trigger overeating; how those with sex addiction can set "safe" borders; and how to set up "lifelines" to prevent relapses.[3] I introduce PAID — Post-Addiction Image Disorder — to help those of you who've worked through your issues to come to terms with who you are post-recovery: your different physical appearance, your possible health problems from former substance abuse, and your loss of familiar defences and old habits.

Self-help books have, in many ways, supplemented or supplanted our doctors, spiritual advisors, friends, and relatives as confidants. In *Food, Sex, and You*, I use my own hard-won experience, plus my knowledge as a therapist specializing in addiction, to guide you toward becoming your healthiest, happiest, most liberated self. It's my hope that the lessons this book contains, told through the stories of real people, along with my practical advice as a therapist, will support you on a daily basis and stay with you for life.[4]

PART I

ADDICTION

The definition of insanity is doing the same thing over and over again and expecting different results.
— Albert Einstein

CHAPTER 1

PERFECTLY BEAUTIFUL: THE IMPOSSIBLE DREAM

When I was five, a checkout clerk at the grocery store said to my mother, "What a beautiful child! You're never going to be able to keep the boys away from her when she grows up."

Afterward, my mother told me, with great intensity, "I want you to know you're more than just your beauty, and you'll always be more than just your beauty. Make sure men know that you're also smart!" Though it would be years before I understood what my mother meant, her fierceness indelibly imprinted her words on my soul.

I received an entirely different kind of message from my father. When I was eight, and going through an ugly stage with braces on my teeth and a bad haircut, I overheard him ask my mother in a worried tone, "Do you think Stacey still has time to become beautiful?"

His question devastated me, and while my parents' messages seemed to conflict, the crux of both was the same: As a girl, beauty would be crucial in defining my life.

I grew up in Thornhill, a suburb of Toronto, in a spacious house with a big backyard, which was the norm in our community. Both sides of my family are Jewish, with a mixed Romanian, Czech, and Polish heritage. My father was a salesman in a men's clothing store, and later the manager for a car dealership. My mother kept house for what would become a family of three girls.

Like many men of his age and background, my father felt that, as the breadwinner, he was entitled to do what he wanted. Though my mother was, and is, a beautiful woman, she lacked confidence as a young wife. I have a vivid memory of standing with her at our back door, watching my father play baseball. My mother was crying because she had no life outside of making meals and washing diapers. The fact that my mother's parents were Holocaust survivors had cast a dark shadow over her upbringing. Security through money was very important, and whenever we were at our grandparents', we weren't allowed to waste food or even use an extra piece of toilet paper. For my mother, personal freedom was what a woman traded for the financial protection of marriage.

That traditional idea of women as the servants of men stayed with me for a long time. It was gratifying to see my mother eventually come into her own power and create a far better balance in her relationship with my father.

Because I spent the first five years of my life as an only child, any early tensions between my mother and father were filtered through me so that I came to feel that I had no childhood. Then came my two younger sisters, Jessica and Melysa.

My father is a good-looking man, six feet with a strong build, sharp features, a moustache, and greying thick, dark hair. As a clothing salesman, he had a keen eye for appearances. I can remember walking with him through malls in Florida, where we vacationed every year, while he rated women from one to ten on their figures, encouraging me to do the same. Though this was supposed to be a game, I was left with the sinking feeling that, as Daddy's little girl, I would never be able to measure up to his or other men's standards.

My father's habit of rating women in cahoots with me as a preadolescent may seem over the top, but he was simply expressing aloud what North American society teaches: that we women will always be judged according to an unattainable physical standard, and that the closer we are to that ideal, the more power we will have.

My body developed early. By age nine I was menstruating, wearing a bra, and already at my full height of five foot six — a giant in my class. Fortunately, that was considered cool, but it did set me apart. By twelve, I was fixated on my body, reading every book and magazine on food, diet, and exercise that I could lay my hands on. I remember seeing a Foot Locker commercial featuring a beautiful blonde with a perfect body, and asking myself, *Can I ever be that? What will it take?* I dreamt about that Foot Locker girl for years. Her body — her perfection — was my goal.

Because I looked mature for my age, I was able to lie my way into a membership at a YMCA gym intended for those sixteen and over. Each day after school, I would grab a bus to go there so I could spend a couple of hours in the weight room. Everyone bought my story about being sixteen, and my new friends at the Y taught me body-building techniques and about the benefits of various diet pills.

My father was a yo-yo dieter. Though he talked about the value of eating proper meals, I would see him drastically restrict his food, then binge on muffins and cake, and go to Dairy Queen to eat Blizzards. He would gain eighty pounds, then lose it, then gain it back. This is what I witnessed my whole life, and I started to do the same. Losing the extra weight was pure torture, and at night I used to break out in a cold sweat because of what I was forcing my body to endure. The bingeing, which I had in common with my father, had come to represent shared love. I was hooked.

I was different from my dad in one important way: When he was at his heaviest, he didn't seem to care what anyone thought, whereas when I was overweight, I felt ashamed of my body and didn't want to be seen. Again, the message indelibly imprinted on my psyche was one largely endorsed by Western culture: As a macho guy, he was entitled to pass judgment on women, whereas I was just a girl struggling to live up to that Foot Locker ideal. He could have his cake and eat it, too. I could not.

I know that my parents loved me dearly, and certainly I loved them. My mother was nurturing and wise, and my dad was so much fun and so great in many ways, but by the time I was twelve, the foundation for the food addiction that would rule my life for two decades had already been laid.

As a product of Western culture, I was hardly alone in my anxieties. Instilling insecurity in women over their physical appearance is the basic strategy used by cosmetics manufacturers, fashion designers, and weight-loss clinics to sell their products, with the mainstream media wildly complicit. Not only do popular magazines bombard us with images of celebrities and models chosen for their beauty, but these images are digitally altered so that celebrity legs are as impossibly long and slender, waists are as wispy, and breasts are as uplifted and enlarged as those of the Barbie dolls we played with as children. Wrinkles are non-existent and skin is glowing.

The "cover" for this once-secret process was blown when *Esquire* magazine featured Michelle Pfeiffer, hailed as one of the world's most beautiful women, on the cover of a 1990 issue with the caption, "What Michelle Pfeiffer Needs ... Is Absolutely Nothing." Subsequently, *Adbusters* obtained and printed a copy of an *Esquire* editorial memo detailing the $1,525 in touch-ups editors deemed necessary before Pfeiffer was fit to be seen by their readers. "Clean up complexion, soften eye lines, soften smile line, add color to lips, trim chin, remove neck lines, soften line under ear lobe ... remove stray hair ... adjust color and add hair on top of head ... add dress on side to create better line ..."

Some editors blame the stars and their publicists for insisting that these alterations be made in order to enhance the stars' image. This could not be said of Kate Winslet, who famously complained that in photographs in a 2003 British edition of *GQ*, editors had excessively slimmed her body to reflect their view of what they thought she *should* look like. As she indignantly exclaimed, "They reduced the size of my legs by about a third!"

In another move that delighted feminists, forty-three-year-old Jamie Lee Curtis posed in a 2002 issue of *More* magazine with no makeup, in harsh light, wearing only a sports bra and panties. This was paired with a contrasting glamour photo of Curtis that had required thirteen people three hours to prepare. As she explained, "I don't have great thighs. I have very big breasts and a soft, fatty little tummy. And I've got back fat." Curtis admitted that she gained the courage to mock her movie-star image through her drug-addiction recovery program. She had become hooked on painkillers as a result of cosmetic eye surgery when she was thirty-five. "I've had a little plastic surgery. I've had a little lipo. I've had a little Botox. And you know what? None of it works. None of it."

More recently, Oscar winner Jennifer Lawrence said about the image of her used in a Miss Dior campaign, "That doesn't look like me at all. People don't look like that!" Her fans vigorously protested when "before" and "after" photos of her for a *Flare* magazine cover revealed that touch-up artists had changed her hairline, hollowed her cheeks, stretched her neck, and thinned her arms and her already slender body. "You look how you look," commented Lawrence. "What are you going to do? Be hungry every single day to make other people happy? That's just dumb."

In 2009, the French version of *Elle* magazine pioneered what came to be called the "raw-celebrity movement" by featuring cover models without makeup or digital touch-ups. Since then, supermarket tabloids have inverted this concept through "gotcha" photography that catches celebrities off guard: "Who's Got the Worst Cellulite in Hollywood?" and "Beach Bodies — Too Fat! Too Thin!" and "Caught Without Their Make-up!" Some editors have even been accused of adding fat and wrinkles to celebrity photos instead of wiping them out.

Even the world's most powerful women can't escape the relentless scrutiny of them as aesthetic objects. When Hillary Clinton was running for the Democratic presidential nomination in 2008, the media seemed to pay as much critical attention to her clothes and hairstyle as to her policies, even predicting that she could become America's first "Pantsuit President." Political buttons, describing Clinton as "2 Fat Thighs, 2 Small Breasts," indicated what could be in store for her now that she is running for the 2016 nomination.

During Germany's last federal election, Chancellor Angela Merkel's proven political savvy didn't keep media louts from peering critically down her cleavage, or bloggers from referring to her "attractiveness gap."

Along with the ideal-beauty standards set by our culture, today's youth have grown up with the technology and the know-how to turn the spotlight on themselves, their friends, and their enemies. From cell-phone cameras to Facebook, from Twitter to Tumblr, they post images of themselves, despite having deep underlying insecurities. How eagerly they count up their Facebook "likes" in search of validation, and how painfully they suffer from mean, anonymous comments that shatter their self-confidence. Their own actions create a vicious circle, because the more eyes that are upon them, the more difficult it is for them to balance their anxieties against their need for recognition. Small wonder that women seek liposuction, tummy tucks, breast implants, and fillers like Juvederm at a younger and younger age. Whereas 1950s housewives invited the neighbours to Tupperware parties, today's career women and socialites stage more fashionable Botox parties, where group-priced injections are served up with the canapés and champagne.

Although beauty is something for which we women have been taught to strive, those born with spectacular looks often discover that their good fortune can have a downside. While men pursue them as sex objects and trophies, other women isolate them because they feel jealous or intimidated. No one truly knows them, and anyone who lives in a vacuum cannot know herself.

Like wealthy or powerful men, beautiful women often find it challenging to sort out the sycophants and the opportunists from those who genuinely admire, like, and love them. However, a critical difference is that women are most sought after when they are young and vulnerable, which is also the time when they are least able to deal with the admiration and jealousy projected upon them, or to benefit from the opportunities that come their way. Too often they learn to depend on their beauty while their more authentic selves shrivel inside.

My client Jennifer was one of those blessed and cursed with beauty. Though a gorgeous, drop-dead blonde, she was, in her view, never perfect enough — a mindset that was becoming increasingly problematic with age.

Jennifer was only thirty-five when she came to see me, but already she had had her nose and her breasts reconstructed, her tummy tucked, and her thighs liposuctioned. Her forehead was regularly frozen with Botox and her expression lines were plumped up with commercial fillers.

Along with an addiction to plastic surgery, Jennifer had a serious eating disorder, an alcohol addiction, a heavy shopping addiction, and a sex and love addiction. A divorcee with three children, she was also deep in denial about her problems, with no idea of who she was or how to climb out of the desperate emotional pit into which she had fallen.

Jennifer remembered obsessing over her weight as early as age ten, smoking at twelve, abusing laxatives at thirteen, and taking diet pills at fifteen. She had grown up in a family in which her father was abusive to her mother, while her mother was abusive to Jennifer. After her father left for another woman, Jennifer's mother conscripted Jennifer, dressed up like a little doll, in her search for a wealthy new husband. Jennifer's early modelling career also exposed her to excessive anxiety about her face and figure.

Though I discovered Jennifer to be an intelligent and witty woman, her looks were all that she believed in. Without that familiar weapon and shield, she felt herself to be powerless. For the past year, Jennifer and I have been working through her hurts and resentments, bringing to light the unhappy childhood patterns that she unconsciously recreated as an adult, and discovering the beauty and strength that she carries inside of her. It's a slow but empowering process, and it's helping her to feel safe, accepted, and loved — not only by herself, but also by the others to whom she is now reaching out.

Marilyn Monroe retained her iconic status as a beauty by dying young and tragically. For Hollywood stars who live a normal lifespan, aging in the limelight can seem especially cruel, which is why so many become reclusive.

As Ava Gardner, a mega-star of the fifties, stated in *Ava Gardner: The Secret Conversations*, by Peter Evans: "Elizabeth Taylor is not beautiful, she is pretty. I was beautiful.... Actors get older. Actresses get old. Life doesn't stop because you're no longer a beauty, or desirable. You just have to make adjustments. Although I'd be lying to you if I told you that losing my looks is no big deal. It hurts, goddamn it, it hurts like a sonofabitch."

CHAPTER 2

FOOD TO BURN: BINGEING AND PURGING

I was seventeen and still living at home when I was forced to recognize that I had an out-of-control bingeing problem. It started so innocently. One day, after eating mamaliga, my favourite Romanian dish, made of cornmeal, butter, and cheese, I still felt hungry, so I made it again. And again. And again. I cooked that dish nine times, and ate every mouthful, aware of the insanity but unable to stop. Afterward, I was so stuffed I could barely climb the stairs to my room, where I lay in bed crying, convinced that something must be terribly wrong with my brain. I kept up this bingeing for three weeks, until I'd ballooned from a slender 118 pounds to a bloated 148.

At this time in my life, I was undergoing scary psychological changes that had deep roots. At age five, I'd been diagnosed with a comprehension problem, and though I'd managed to pass each grade, fitting into the education system was always a struggle. I excelled at sports, like running and gymnastics, and eventually developed the social skills to make friends. However, I still felt like a misfit since I didn't experiment with drugs and sex like the other kids were doing. My mother had lectured me from an early age about the importance of keeping my virginity. Only girls who were perfect and untouched, she warned, made the best candidates in the all-important marriage sweepstakes.

Of course, by then I was aware that men found me attractive. I thrived on their attention and worked hard on my external shell, because without the assurance that it gave me, I really didn't know who I was. I always had a boyfriend who was older than my high-school friends, but my fear was much stronger than my hormones or my curiosity, so sex remained off-limits.

At age seventeen, I met Neil while on a double date. As soon as we started seeing each other, I knew we would get married. I knew this partly because I'm intuitive and partly because Neil was exactly the kind of man for whom I had been looking. Four years older than me, he was tall, dark, and very handsome, professionally established, and a good person. Though I suspected that he regarded me as some kind of trophy, that didn't disturb me. *Wasn't that what I was supposed to be?*

Perhaps it was my fear of physical intimacy with Neil, or the pressures of being the perfect mate in preparation for our perfect life together that had triggered my binge on Romanian mamaliga. I was used to overeating, then restricting and exercising, but in the past I'd always been able to keep a tenuous balance. Now, I was bursting with an extra thirty pounds. When Neil invited me to a friend's engagement party, I was as incapable of leaving my house as if I had been shackled to the bedpost, even though I desperately wanted to attend.

Neil was understanding. "Just do what you need to do to look after this." I knew deep down that there was a problem, but I didn't want to face how serious it was. Bingeing then severely restricting my diet at times seemed just normal — after all, I had learned this behaviour from my father while growing up. At other times I thought maybe I had a chemical imbalance. Perhaps my brain didn't tell my stomach when I was hungry, or my stomach didn't tell my brain when it was full, so there was a disconnect? At other times I fooled myself into thinking this was the way that health-conscious people acted, and that what I was doing showed willpower and strength. I did not see my problem with food for what it was: unhealthy and out-of-control cyclical behaviour. My obsession with food and weight had controlled my entire life.

At first I believed that I could get things under control, but the harder I tried, the worse my problem — and the greater my shame — became. I really couldn't understand why I couldn't enjoy food like "normal" people. I'd watch them eat full meals yet manage to stay slim, and I'd ask myself, What's wrong with me? Why do I have to suffer so pointlessly?

I fell into a deep depression, during which I dreaded every meal, terrified to eat anything in case one innocuous mouthful, needed to nourish my body, started a week of mindless, trance-like bingeing, in which I could not feel myself as myself from one moment to the next. I begged my mother and father, "Please — I need help!"

They agreed that I should see a psychiatrist, so I made an appointment with one connected to a local hospital. We'd spoken for less than fifteen minutes before the doctor prescribed a drug for me: Zoloft. Known as an SSRI, which stands for "selective serotonin reuptake inhibitor," it is designed to treat depression, anxiety, and obsessive-compulsive disorder.

Though I felt the psychiatrist didn't understand me, I was filled with hope. At last, something was going to take away my pain!

In fairness, she did warn me. "Don't see Zoloft as a solution to your emotional and mental problems. Work on them as well."

What did she mean? I didn't know, or want to know. Though now I much prefer naturopathic medicine, back then I went for the conventional. My overriding feeling was, Why would anyone choose to be unhappy if there is something that can help?

In fact, Zoloft did work like magic. After I'd gained and lost that same thirty pounds a few times more, the drug kicked in, and I stopped bingeing, which allowed me to maintain a "skinny weight" of 120 pounds. For the first time in a long while, I had a life.

Despite my newfound confidence, I still felt like Neil's doll, who dressed and acted in the way he had taught me. I remember him exclaiming once in exasperation, "Where is your voice?" He wanted me to speak up, but I didn't know how.

That began to change when Neil went on vacations with his buddies, leaving me alone. I started to demand more of him. I became more real, and therefore more attractive. I think that's when Neil began to fall genuinely and deeply in love with me.

After we got engaged, Neil and I bought a house in Thornhill. Because I was still afraid of my body, it took a while before I let myself become intimate with him. Everything about this relationship was a learning experience for me; however, after a year of living together, I felt ready to launch our new life. We set a date for our wedding.

Of course, this meant having the perfect wedding. The Zoloft provided some normalcy and helped me to regulate my binges, allowing me to fit into my poofy white dress, which I wore with a tiara. We had about five hundred guests, which was part of the wedding's overkill. Our parents had given us a spectacle, whereas I probably would have been happier with something smaller. Everyone seemed to have a good time, and the event lived up to my image of perfection. Now, at twenty-two, I was eager to leave behind my shameful, hurtful problems and simply enjoy my perfect life.

As Neil's wife, I had a ready-made role in our Thornhill community. The peaceful sense of normalcy granted me by Zoloft lasted two years, with low libido as a side effect. That seemed like a fair trade-off to me, since I wasn't used to a lusty sex life, but it was frustrating for Neil.

As young marrieds, Neil and I partied with a wealthy crowd that drank a lot and used marijuana. When I'd first smoked a joint at nineteen in Amsterdam, I had laughed hysterically, experienced hallucinations, lost my inhibitions, and become extremely hungry. Despite these intriguing effects, I hadn't tried it again for another three years. That's when I began to smoke joints to go along with our crowd. Since alcohol had never been a problem for me, I was sure I could control my marijuana use, but I was having so much fun that I became addicted, failing to realize that the drug was counteractive to Zoloft, my SSRI medication.

Just as in Amsterdam, I would get ferociously hungry while coming down from a high, so I would binge because food tasted so delicious. I had always liked yogurt, but with marijuana it tasted like yogurt on steroids. Then, the next morning, I would have the largest food hangover. I would sweat for days while my body attempted to regulate itself, after which I would either continue to binge or starve myself. I would exercise beyond total exhaustion even when my body felt it couldn't stand another push-up. I would take a laxative or swallow diet pills. I would read diet magazines and plan new diets, because I still didn't understand that something external could not cure what was an emotional and mental disorder.

Since the Zoloft was no longer working, I stopped taking it. Like other addicts in denial, I refused to blame the marijuana for my bingeing, and since I could still control my weight by drastic means, I was able to pretend to the outside world that everything was normal.

When the fun of the marijuana wore off, I became lethargic. I started to wear the same clothes every day and to stop caring for myself. With my defences crumbling, it was now just me and the bingeing, and that was when depression really set in. I began to fear that I would end up weighing three hundred pounds, which was terrifying for someone who was also addicted to perfection.

Fooling everyone, including myself, was getting harder. It was a shock when an aunt, who caught me while I was out shopping, asked if I was pregnant. I'm proud that I at least had the courage to snap back, "No, I'm not pregnant. I'm sick. I'm a binge eater."

I didn't really care what my aunt thought about me. What controlled me was what I thought about myself, because I wasn't comfortable in my own skin, regardless of whether I was thin or fat. Even when people complimented me in the most amazing way, I never believed them, because I didn't like myself at all.

Unlike other addictive substances, food isn't one you can give up. There was always grocery shopping, meal preparation, and entertaining to keep me in touch with the enemy. My obsession made me a great cook; I knew exactly where to buy each item and how to prepare and serve it. I also knew how to hide it. I had married the right man, because Neil was well-grounded and stood by me in my confusion but also turned a blind eye to my behaviour because he didn't want to find fault with me. The fact that he travelled a great deal made my deceptions easier.

I now know that addiction is a way of creating a distraction to keep us from facing something deep and painful in our lives. I had everything I had always thought I wanted — how could I *not* be happy? Today, as a therapist, I often meet people who are desperate like I was, whose lives should be full of joy but who are blinded by their disease to everything good about themselves. My illness lied to me. Addiction always lies, and as long as I believed those lies, it was always stronger than I was. I had almost every symptom I would later use to diagnose my clients' eating disorders:

- Obsessively self-critical about weight and body image
- Obsessive thoughts of food
- Obsessive food restriction
- Obsessive calorie-counting
- Obsessive exercising
- Unable to separate hunger from desire, obsessively bingeing as a result
- Use of food to numb or deal with emotions
- Fear of certain foods because of weight gain
- Frequent checking of body weight
- Trouble maintaining a body weight that is normal for age and height
- Misuse/abuse of laxatives, diuretics, or enemas
- Hoarding high-calorie foods
- Eating alone, in secret, or late at night

Despite all the evidence, I couldn't see beyond my issues with food to my addiction to marijuana, and I couldn't see beyond my addiction to marijuana to my underlying emotional and mental problems. I was sliding into what I would later describe as my suck hole — a big black pit filled with mud and quicksand.

Every day was clouded by guilt and shame, thanks to the lie that refused to allow me to take credit for my successes or to enjoy events that should have made me happy. I had clothes in my closet from size zero to size twelve, and even when I could squeeze into a favourite size-one outfit, I couldn't enjoy an evening out because I was already planning what food I would binge on when I got home.

I was still too far down in my suck hole to ask myself, Okay, Stacey, now WHAT IS EATING YOU?

The day in 2000 that I found out I was pregnant, I quit marijuana, cold turkey, along with cigarettes and alcohol. I knew those things would be terrible for the fetus, and at least I had enough willpower and maternal instinct to want to protect my baby from my addictions. I had no trouble kicking the cigarettes, and alcohol had never been a problem, but despite the claim of many people that marijuana is non-addictive, coming off of it was tough. For a while, I would dream so vividly that I had smoked a joint that when I awoke in the morning, I would have difficulty understanding it was only a dream. That's how bad my addiction had been. I get shivers even now just thinking about it.

Getting pregnant had started out as yet another distraction for me. All my friends were having babies. Neil wanted a baby. I needed something meaningful to fill my days. Pregnancy was a legitimate reason for gaining weight, and the script in my head called for my having three kids before I was thirty.

Without the relief provided by marijuana, my bingeing grew worse. I was eating non-stop, but because my new motivation was to have a healthy baby, this no longer seemed like bingeing. I completely let my body go, figuring that gaining weight was part of a natural process and that I would lose all the excess poundage when I gave birth. I'd always been most critical of my midsection, so seeing it expand was my worst nightmare playing out in reality, but wasn't I supposed to be getting fat? I'd been abusing my body for so long that all I knew was either starving or bingeing, and I didn't dare starve because I was so afraid of harming my baby.

I ate until I weighed two hundred pounds — a gain of eighty-five pounds. Now I was heavier than my husband, which was really scary. When my father joked that I was a Hoover vacuum cleaner, sucking up any food that wasn't nailed to the table, I shouted at him to leave the house and never return — the first time I'd ever stood up to my dad. Though that was my hormones lashing out, this incident succeeded in shifting our relationship in a positive way.

At eight months, my body broke out in a massive rash — something else I couldn't control. I had sciatica, which is a painful condition caused by compression of the spinal nerves, and it led to weakness in my legs, so that I would keel over for no apparent reason.

One terrible afternoon, I locked myself in my car and blared Def Leppard and AC/DC hard rock. I must have been really desperate. I was eager to have my baby — pregnancy had been my choice — but I wasn't emotionally ready because of my unresolved problems and that led to a mess of confusing responses.

My labour was mercifully short but very painful. I had been dilated to four centimetres for a month, so the birth happened too quickly for the nurses to administer an epidural to block my pain. After a traumatic ninety minutes, during which I thought I would die, I gave birth to my beautiful son on December 19, 2000.

Tyler wasn't a happy camper. I wish I'd known when I was playing Def Leppard and AC/DC that a child's emotions are formed while in the womb. He was so colicky that I spent the next six months travelling from doctor to doctor — for him, for me —and that became my whole life. I would be up all night, then Neil would go to work the next morning, leaving me with a troubled baby and a spinning head. My self-worth was so dependent on being pretty and skinny that the extra weight I was still carrying meant, in my mind, that I had nothing to offer anyone. I couldn't find my place in my own life. I wanted to jump out a window.

Once I stopped breastfeeding, I started smoking marijuana every night after putting the baby to bed. That was when a friend told me about a great diet: "Don't eat carbs. They're poison." That clicked for me. All I had to do to lose my pregnancy poundage was to eliminate carbs. In fact, that's what did happen, and it was the worst result possible, because now I was sure I had the magic key to control my weight forever.

When cutting carbs no longer balanced my bingeing, I learned to drop ten pounds in five days by eating only egg whites with water, taking laxatives, and over-exercising. I had every diet pill ever manufactured, and while vacationing in Mexico, I was able to buy weight-loss drugs I couldn't get in Canada. The adrenalin of starvation created a false high, so that I felt like I could climb the CN Tower in five seconds. Because of weight loss, I was seeing parts of my body I hadn't seen before. I could feel the bones of my hips rubbing on my mattress at night, and when I awoke, my hips were numb and bruised from the pressure. That's how skinny I was. I had a little scale for weighing my food and a notebook in which I obsessively calculated calories. If I ate so much as a lettuce leaf, I wrote that down. I was on the bathroom scale forty times a day. My entire life revolved around food and my weight.

One part of my body proved beyond my power to fix through exercise and diet. Before my pregnancy, I had had full B-cup breasts that were naturally high-set — the only thing about my body that I truly loved. During the four months that I was breastfeeding, I had so much milk that the nurses told me I was the luckiest woman in the world — I could sell it on the street like gold!

Being excessive as always, I took to pumping my breast milk, then bagging and freezing the milk so that my kid would never be without. At one point, I must have had about forty bags in the freezer — enough to feed a whole ward of babies!

But my obsessive pumping destroyed the tissue in my breasts, so that they flopped on my chest like deflated and shrivelled beanbags. I resisted plastic surgery because my mother was dead set against it, and because of my own fear of surgical complications, along with concerns about the further stretching of my skin by implants.

Instead, I bought the biggest bra that I could find at Victoria's Secret, then stuffed it with the gel implants used by women who have had mastectomies. My old clothes wouldn't fit, and I couldn't leave the house without the gels, because I couldn't suddenly go from double-Ds to flat. I spent days trying to figure out how to fit the gels into a dress that was backless, because I couldn't wear a bra with it. Bathing suits were the worst. Hard as this may be for others to understand, I still didn't think that I had a problem beyond how I might look at the beach the next day.

Not surprisingly, it was four years before I wanted to get pregnant again. Since I knew what to expect, I handled this pregnancy much better than the first with regard to food and exercise, but I still gained eighty-five pounds. It took me seven months to lose that extra weight — longer than after the first pregnancy — and I wasn't able to become as skinny as before. I had given up cigarettes and marijuana for this pregnancy as well, and when it was over, I vowed, *Never again!*

Though I was a caring and engaged mother, my demons remained in charge of much of my life. I would plan binges days in advance, and then, when the coast was clear, I would go shopping, maybe to six different food markets, because one had a certain chocolate sauce, another had my favourite ice cream, and another had the Oreo cookies and peanut butter I craved. Then I would hide these things all over the house — the chocolate sauce in the microwave, the peanut butter in a closet, the cookies in the basement, the ice cream stashed in the back of the freezer. Though secrecy protected my addiction, it also served another purpose: to protect my children. As the person responsible for their nutrition, I was adamant about not passing my obsessions on to them.

Always after my bingeing came the necessary restricting, the laxatives, and the exhaustive exercise. When lunching with friends, I was limited to only a few restaurants that had food low enough in calories to fit my diet, and sometimes I brought my lunch in a bag. Not surprisingly, my friends became tired of hearing me complain about my weight — I was like a black cloud hanging over everyone. Though I felt like I was drowning, I didn't know any way to deal with stress besides gorging and restricting, which of course created greater stress, spinning me in a vicious circle. At my worst I wondered, Could I really be possessed by demons? Why else would I act so insanely?

When I tried to convince my mother that I was sick, she would say, "You don't have any problems except those you make for yourself."

One day my grandmother took me aside and said, "I'm going to tell you a story."

She described what she and her other family members had endured during the Holocaust, including what had happened to one of her sisters, who'd had something done to her sexual organs so that she couldn't have children.

That severe emotional shakedown put my struggle in perspective, flipping a switch inside my head and helping me to move forward. I asked myself: What am I doing, wasting the best years of my life? When I'm eighty or ninety, I'll realize that my body was never going to be better than it was now.

I started to look around myself with open, anguished eyes. Friends my age were acquiring a great education or building their careers. My sisters were enthusiastic about testing their talents as artists. I had a neighbour who seemed thrilled by the privilege of taking care of her husband and two sons, and whenever I looked into her radiant face, I asked myself, Where did my happiness go? I remembered having had it in the past, and seeing happiness in others made me want mine back.

I had already tried a couple of jobs — co-owner of a gift shop and makeup artist. I'd even earned my real-estate licence during my second pregnancy in 2004, hoping to be as successful at selling houses as my mother was, but I could never persuade myself to use it. Apart from looking after my family, all I did was work out at the gym, shop, lunch with friends, and obsess over food. From the outside, I appeared to be leading a fantasy life, but to me it felt purposeless and pointless.

When I searched for someone to blame for my depression, I didn't have far to look. My husband had a great career and often travelled to exciting places for business, stirring up my resentment even more. I knew I wasn't cut out to live in the shadow of someone else's dream, and I hated being dependent on him for money. The more I thought about it, the more my warped mind convinced me that Neil's success was at fault for my lost ambition.

I had vowed I would never lead the life of a disempowered housewife, but here I was, metaphorically crying at the back door, watching my husband enjoy an independent life. I'm not sure if I would have felt elated to know that one day I, too, would have a purposeful life that challenged and thrilled me, or if I would have felt suicidal to know that getting there would take several more years of hell.

PART II

RECOVERY

If you plan on being anything less than you are capable of
being, you will probably be unhappy all the days of your life.
— Abraham Maslow

CHAPTER 3

OVEREATERS ANONYMOUS: ABOARD THE LIFE RAFT

I was thirty in 2005 when I joined Overeaters Anonymous, which is run on the same principles as Alcoholic Anonymous and has chapters worldwide.

A friend who was struggling with the same weighty issues understood what I was going through and suggested that I attend a meeting with her. She chose a meeting that would be the "strongest," meaning that its members would have the most recovery time to their credit. The group's coordinator had warned her that we would be hearing a lot about "God" and a "higher power," even though OA is not affiliated with any specific religion. Since all I wanted was to lose weight, and OA seemed to offer a platform for confessionals rather than a diet program, I was skeptical, yet desperate enough to try anything. *How had I become so humbled that I was willing to share my shame with strangers?* At least hearing the success stories of others might prove inspirational.

This meeting was held at a local church, and I remember very clearly how uncomfortable I felt walking up to the door that day, not knowing what to expect but determined not to bolt. After being welcomed by a volunteer, my friend and I sat quietly, along with a hundred others. Many were very heavy, and I weighed only 140 pounds at the time. I could see them looking at me, and maybe wondering, *What's she doing here?* That seemed like a good question. *What* was *I doing there?* At the same time, I felt anticipation. Perhaps I would find a piece of a solution at this meeting.

The volunteer who was leading the group that day asked each of us newcomers to introduce ourselves by our first name. I managed to choke out the words, "I'm Stacey, and I'm a compulsive overeater."

The group then recited the Serenity Prayer: "God grant me the serenity to accept the things I cannot change, the courage to change the things I can, and the wisdom to know the difference. Thy will, not mine, be done."

Various members read passages from a big book entitled *Alcoholics Anonymous.* That confused me. *Why are we reading about alcohol? That's never been my problem.* I turned to my friend with a questioning look. *Have we come to the wrong meeting?* But no, the readers were substituting the word *food* for the word *alcohol.*

The leader awarded medals to those who had achieved a certain amount of abstinence. Again I wondered, How can you abstain from food? When I listened more carefully, I discovered that these medals were not awarded for adherence to rigid rules, but rather for the meeting of goals established between members and their sponsors. The medals recognized members' weeks, or months, or years of recovery. I also discovered that lapsing even once meant losing all your recovery time, which seemed harsh, since to me "recovery" still meant not dying from overeating.

We listened to more readings from a second book that was passed around in the circle. This book dealt specifically with overeating. The thoughts expressed — *letting go, surrendering, forgiveness, humility, spirituality* — were ones my mind had never before encompassed in connection with my addiction. I wondered, Did other newcomers feel the same as I did, or was I the only one who would prove too stupid to recover? I was sure that my eating disorder was worse than anyone else's in this room. I was sure no one had suffered as much as I had, or could begin to understand what I'd been through.

After the readings, we newcomers were invited to listen while those who had at least one week of recovery told their stories. I sat shocked and spellbound to hear a part of my story in the account of every single person. It both scared and relieved me to know that so many others were like me, but not exactly like me. I could relate to every person, both male and female, as if each were a facet of me.

At the end of the formal meeting, a collection tray was passed around for donations, but no fee was charged.

We newbies were then paired with volunteers to talk in private about our individual situations. When my volunteer asked for my response to what I had observed, I replied truthfully, "I feel hopeful and skeptical."

She nodded. "Yes, but you should come to six meetings before deciding this program is not for you. For it to work, you must ask someone to be your sponsor, then follow whatever plan the two of you decide upon. You must also commit to attending two or three meetings every week."

This volunteer had seven years of abstinence behind her. Seven years! I could barely make it through a couple of days without bingeing. I desperately wanted what she had, so I committed on the spot. "Will you sponsor me?"

She was reluctant. "I'm already sponsoring four others."

I begged her, because I knew intuitively that she was my messenger.

She agreed to take me on.

For the next three years, from 2005 to 2008, I attended at least three OA meetings a week. I struggled to understand that in order for me to be free of my food addiction or binge eating, I would have to refrain from eating the foods that I binged on and that I would have to come to a meeting a minimum of three times a week. I struggled against the thought that this was to be a permanent way of life for me. I struggled against the idea that I would have to give up forever all the foods I loved. I struggled against my ingrained belief that I would never achieve the weight and figure that I still wanted. I struggled to understand why I couldn't reach the goals others were attaining.

Every failure or success was an excuse to binge. Someone would honk at me at a stoplight, and I'd binge in anger. Someone would compliment me on a dress, and I'd binge in celebration. Someone would make a remark that seemed slighting, and I'd binge in resentment, then spend another few hours blaming that person for my depression, which caused me to binge some more. Sometimes I was so discouraged by my abject failure that I'd rush home from an OA meeting to devour a tub of ice cream with chocolate and peanut butter. Then I'd call or email my sponsor to complain that the program wasn't working for me. She'd reply that the program always works, and that if I kept coming back, the miracle would happen for me as it had for so many others. It was, she insisted, a matter of faith.

My sponsor was an angel of patience, but she could also be very hard on me. She kept repeating that addiction is a disease that always lies. She told me that every addict has two brains. One is your true self — the part of you that is without an addiction. The other belongs completely to the disease. When this addicted brain takes over, it convinces you that it's okay to have one piece of cake, even if you know that you will end up eating the whole thing.

For the first eight months of OA meetings, I was too terrified to say anything other than my declaration, "Hi, I'm Stacey, and I'm a compulsive overeater." Finally, I did work up the courage to share a bit of my struggle and caused several startled members to exclaim, "Oh, so you do have a voice!"

By then, I'd heard stories that were worse than mine, as well as stories of almost miraculous recovery. Some of those successful people weren't skinny, but they seemed so happy. I ran around asking them how they'd achieved their miracles until a woman with twenty years of recovery replied, "No matter how many people you ask, or who they are, or what their qualifications, only you can choose to stop the insanity."

Choose? What did that mean? Did I really have power over my addict's conniving brain?

Like Alcoholics Anonymous, Overeaters Anonymous works on the basis of a twelve-step program:

> **Step 1:** I admit that I am powerless over my disease and my life has become unmanageable.

That is the most important step, and the hardest for me. Though I'd failed in my struggle to control my addiction, I didn't see how turning myself into a helpless victim was going to improve my situation. It took me quite a while to understand that, paradoxically, admitting to the problem and surrendering my futile attempts to control it was the first step toward genuinely empowering myself by reaching out and up. Like my grandparents who made it through the Holocaust, I wanted to be a survivor.

> **Step 2:** I accept that there is a higher power much greater than myself that will guide and help me, and I surrender myself to that power.

Being Jewish, I wasn't supposed to get down on my knees to pray, but that's what my sponsor told me to do, so that's what I did. I prayed to this unknown higher power to take away my insanity. I did this religiously, like it was a job.

> **Step 3:** I will turn over my will and my life to the care of God, as I personally understand God to be.

Though still uncertain of my faith in the program, I kept those first three steps written out beside my bed, and every morning I'd read and recite them. For me, trusting in the universe came to mean no longer letting the numbers on my scale reflect my worth. It meant seeing myself as more than a physical person by expanding the spirituality that was a natural part of me.

> **Step 4:** I will make a searching and fearless moral inventory of myself.

Wow! Step 4 taught me so much! I began to understand how resentful I was of people whom I envied, in turn drawing their resentment toward me. For the first time, I began to see who I was behind my mask, and it was a revelation.

> **Step 5:** I admit to God, to myself, and to other human beings the exact nature of my faults.

The realization that I was not as perfect as I wanted to be brought with it the realization that I was not as imperfect as I feared. Though I had much work ahead, I had a choice, and a voice, to set myself free to become the person I wanted to be.

> **Step 6:** I am entirely ready and willing to surrender to God to correct my defects of character.

Now, at last, I began to understand the concept of letting go of my frantic efforts at control in order to allow the recovery process to move forward.

> **Step 7:** I humbly ask God to remove my shortcomings.

I came to terms with the fact that I would need outside strength and patience to pursue my goal of recovery as an ongoing journey, and that this new struggle, no matter how difficult, would be better than a life of addiction.

> **Step 8:** I will make a list of all the persons I have harmed and be willing to make amends to them.

This taught me to step outside my shame and guilt to confront specific wrongs, to take responsibility for them, and to ask for forgiveness.

> **Step 9:** I will make direct amends to such people wherever possible, except when doing so would injure them further or harm others.

Direct action required me to face life on terms other than my own, including those of my addiction — and to accept other people's reality.

> **Step 10:** I will continue to take personal inventory, and when I am wrong, to promptly admit it.

This taught me to consciously and continuously monitor myself, and to stop the blame game, both in regard to other people and to my addiction.

Step 11: I will seek through prayer and meditation to improve my conscious contact with God, as I understand this higher power, praying only for knowledge of God's will for me, along with the power to carry this out.

This confirmed, through peaceful connection with the all-powerful universe, my ability to discover my highest purpose as the secret to my recovery while remaining conscious, grounded, and sane.

Step 12: I will practise these principles in all of my affairs because being of service is the greatest gift I can give to myself and another human being.[5]

Through the twelve steps, I would eventually come to a spiritual awakening in which I understood that it was my duty to give back what I had received. Though I was as yet unaware of it, this would mean helping others who suffered addiction as I had. But first, I had to reach a place of relative peace and safety, which was still years up the road, and I had no guarantee that I would ever make it.

As well as working through the twelve steps, I adopted a self-affirmative mantra that I was to say over and over until I believed it: "I love and approve of myself."

My sponsor also helped me to focus more practically on my eating disorder. Since I knew only starving and bingeing, I had to learn, like a baby, how to eat food for hunger, nourishment, and pleasure. The first rule was that I must eat three meals a day and a snack. When my sponsor told me to list all the foods that I binge on, I put almost everything on my list, because everything seemed dangerous.

She then asked me, "What would you order at a restaurant if you weren't afraid of getting fat?"

I replied, "Pasta, bread, and a glass of wine," which was what I often ordered, but without being able to stop at only one portion.

She then asked, "What if you could eat that every night?"

"I would soon be three hundred pounds!"

"How badly do you want to recover?"

"More than anything."

"Enough to *try* anything?"

"Yes."

"Then, why don't you have pasta, bread, and wine every night, while giving yourself over to the universe through the step program? Remember, you must continue to eat three meals a day plus a snack. You may gain or lose five pounds, but eventually your body will arrive at its set point."[6]

I was still afraid. "What if my set point is a high one?"

"Just have faith."

What choice did I have, after all my failures, but to try something different? "Okay, but I'll omit the wine, because I'm only an occasional drinker." Secretly I wondered, How did my sponsor ever achieve seven years of recovery with ideas like these?

I stifled these objections, vowing to have faith in the process. For four months, I ate three meals a day along with a snack. Every night I had pasta and bread for dinner, partly because I was supposed to, but partly because I felt like it. This was new for me, and for a long while it was hard. I'd always eaten out of fear, guilt, and shame, but eventually I really enjoyed the pasta, and knowing I could have it again the next day for dinner, without restricting myself afterward as a punishment, allowed me to feel safe and satisfied when leaving the table.

At the same time, I prayed every morning and every night, asking God to free me from my obsessions, and to allow me to lead a happy, fulfilled life. Each evening I wrote down ten things for which I was grateful. I started a journal, and I repeated my steps and my affirmation. For the first time, I began to feel what it was like to be *in* my body, rather than just to *have* a body. That meant honouring and respecting it, rather than using and abusing it as if detached from it. While I had already been open to my spirituality, OA plugged me into it like I was switching on a light, so that I felt a connection to the universe, both higher up and all around me.

After four months of pasta, I hadn't gained a pound. I still weighed 140. That was shocking to me, but also a little disappointing, because I'd secretly and typically hoped to lose weight.

I began to crave other foods besides pasta, especially protein. By then, my body had learned that it didn't have to hold on to fat for fear it was going to be starved, so when I substituted protein for pasta, I slowly but surely did start to lose weight. For the first time ever, my little stomach pouch, which I thought was genetic, disappeared, and my hormones levelled out. I felt as if I were awakening from a long, deep sleep as I embraced the program 100 percent, and I received back 100 percent. I began to wonder, could this be the beginning of the miracle for which I'd prayed?

Since I was still at a very vulnerable stage, I never left my house until I knew how, where, and when I would get my three meals that day. That sometimes meant preparing and bringing my lunch — a practice that, by the way, I still follow. Because I now knew what my trigger foods were — chocolate, cake, doughnuts, cookies, chips, ice cream, and peanut butter — if I was confronted with these at other people's homes, I'd go to the washroom to say the Serenity Prayer.

Despite all of this success, I was often at odds with my sponsor. After I reported to her what I'd been eating for a few days, or for the week, she would sometimes scold me for reasons that came as a shock to me.

"Stacey, my gut feeling tells me that you're secretly dieting. I find it hard to believe that you went to a restaurant last night, and that all you wanted was steamed vegetables. You lost some weight, and now you want to lose more. Quit it!"

If I was dieting, that was a secret from me as well, because I was still so confused from bingeing and restricting that I didn't understand what "normal" eating for a "normal" appetite meant.

A more serious problem developed between us over my suggestion that I introduce small amounts of the binge foods I loved.

Her adamant response was, "You're an addict! That will never work. You know that if you eat one serving of ice cream, you'll eat the whole tub. You can't be a social eater any more than an alcoholic can be a social drinker."

My rebellious attitude stemmed from the fact that I had been reaching out to other mentors and other programs while still attending OA. I was now seeing a wonderful therapist who seldom talked directly about food, focusing instead on the underlying emotions fuelling my addiction. I was also consulting a doctor who specialized in neurologically based eating disorders, whose philosophy clashed in significant ways with that of OA.

As I see-sawed back and forth between these two mentors, my OA sponsor challenged me to make a choice. I decided to go with the doctor. OA had set my feet firmly on the road to recovery, but I had always struggled with the idea that I would need to remain a lifelong member to sustain my abstinence. In my view, the twelve steps were so ingrained in my soul that attending meetings was no longer necessary. I had taken what I needed from the program, and now it was important for me to move on.

Leaving OA and my sponsor was wrenching for me. She had rocked my world! I had learned so much from her, but even as an OA dropout, the organization's values remain a vital part of my being.

This was proven by an *aha* moment that validated the program's and my sponsor's wisdom.

I remember, so very specifically, walking through the Bayview Village mall, not at my sleekest weight, but dutifully repeating my mantra, *I love and approve of myself. I love and approve of myself.* Though I'd been doing this for years as just another obsessive habit, all of a sudden it struck me on a level that included every cell in my body. Yes, I *do* love and approve of myself! For the first time, I actually *did* believe this. Nothing external had changed. I was just out walking on an ordinary day in an ordinary place, but a significant transformation had taken place inside me that radiates to this day.

Here was my magic moment, just as my sponsor had promised.

No, I wasn't entirely out of the woods, but I had caught a glimpse of the future, and even from where I was standing, it looked very bright.

CHAPTER 4

ADHD:
BINGEING ON MY BRAIN

When I was five, my parents enrolled me in a private Jewish school, where I had to learn Hebrew, read the Torah, and pray for hours. I hated it so much that I would have preferred to have a root canal every day. I couldn't do anything right, and I didn't get along with the other kids, so, yes, I was a troublemaker. I was always being sent to the principal's office, and the teachers used to take away my snack to discipline me — reinforcing, yet again, my idea of food as reward and punishment.

I remember taking my spite out on the smartest, prettiest girl in the class, who always drew nice pictures. I would turn around and scribble on her artwork, driving the teachers ballistic. I wanted to be like her. I wanted to have what she had, and to do what she did, and I couldn't handle my jealousy.

When one of my teachers suggested that I might have a learning disability, my parents took me to a psychologist to be tested, which was unusual for the times. The results determined that I had an undefined comprehension problem.

As part of that testing, the psychologist asked me to make a wish. I remember telling her, "I want my parents to be healthy and safe."

The psychologist was amazed. "Most kids ask for candy or toys. I've never before heard a five-year-old make such a mature wish."

At Hebrew school, I was demoted from the advanced class to the basic class as a result of the testing, confirming my feeling that there was something wrong with me. I didn't think I was stupid, but being labelled "basic" instilled in my subconscious a sense that I would always fail to measure up. Thankfully, educators now know that not every kid fits into the system, and alternative schools do exist. Meanwhile, I was stuck in that Hebrew school until the end of grade two, when my parents enrolled me in Thornhill Public School. Though that better suited me, I still couldn't focus properly, and I still didn't fit in. Getting a good education was never a priority for me. What I fixated on was having a perfect body, which meant fighting my food addiction, and that often left me trembling on the verge of a breakdown.

All these memories flooded back when Dr. Lance Levy, a pediatrician specializing in eating disorders, suggested that I be tested for Attention Deficit Hyperactivity Disorder (I was making progress with my recovery at Overeaters Anonymous at the time). When I had been examined as a child back in 1980, ADHD was not a common diagnosis. Today, 3 to 7 percent of school-aged children are said to have this condition, leading to fears that now it may be over- rather than under-diagnosed.

As soon as I looked through the following list of symptoms supplied by the American Psychiatric Association's *Diagnostic and Statistical Manual of Mental Disorders* (*DSM-IV-TR*), I had no difficulty seeing myself as a child:

- Difficulty paying attention and easily distracted
- Difficulty following instructions and failure to finish tasks
- Difficulty remaining seated, frequently fidgets or squirms
- Difficulty managing emotional responses, leading to temper outbreaks
- Difficulty in dealing with delayed gratification
- Talks excessively, often interrupting others
- Easily frustrated, with frequent mood swings and behavioural inconsistencies
- Daydreams excessively

When Dr. Levy not only confirmed that I had ADHD but also linked this neurologically based psychiatric disorder to my compulsive eating, I was amazed. Despite the many times that I'd felt so out of control that I suspected my brain was out of whack, I had become convinced that I was an emotional eater. Now, I knew my brain had been playing a major role in my unstoppable bingeing. This knowledge opened new doors for treatment. I had always attributed my thoughts to my brain and my emotions to my heart, but now I understood that human behaviour is far more complex than that.

Dr. Levy also explained that ADHD affects women very differently than men. Women often internalize their hyperactivity, manifesting it through restless thoughts, unstable emotions, and irrational obsessions. Though not all of us with ADHD have eating disorders, this link was also confirmed by Dr. Russell Barkley, an international expert on ADHD, in the *New York Times* (February 16, 2013) when he connected ADHD with eating disorders, especially bulimia (induced vomiting), as well as with depression and anxiety in women.

Men, on the other hand, are more likely to express their hyperactivity through antisocial behaviour — compulsive anger, violence, drug addiction, and reckless driving. Because of this acting out, men are usually diagnosed earlier. Women are more commonly diagnosed in their thirties and forties, often when they take a child with problems to a doctor and discover they share some of the same symptoms.

As adults, both men and women with ADHD are likely to be undereducated and underemployed relative to their intellectual ability and family background — once again, a symptom I had no problem acknowledging in myself.

While ADHD can be a lifelong challenge, understanding its symptoms allows for better handling of the problems it creates. For me, knowing that my impulsive, compulsive inability to control my eating had a neurological base as well as an emotional one made me more sympathetic to myself and undercut my guilt and shame. The fact that I now knew my deafness to reason while bingeing was not simply a character flaw strengthened my resolve to avoid foods and situations that might trigger that out-of-control response. It also helped me to know that I was not alone, and that experts understood this dimension of my addiction.

For ADHDers like me, it isn't just compulsiveness that is the enemy, but also our hyperactive lack of patience with the slowness of weight loss. It is those things, along with our black-and-white thinking, that drive us to starve and binge, resulting in frustration when our beleaguered bodies fail to deliver on our unrealistic expectations.

Since we are easily bored, the moment we put down our empty ice-cream bowl, we fixate on something else, like maybe a piece of cake. Starting a new diet that requires us to buy different foods and new supplements feels so promising at first, as does joining a new gym. For a while, fixation on a new relationship or a new job may seem more exciting than food, but eventually even this stirs up a new set of anxieties that loops us back to overeating. Our disappointment in other aspects of life easily collects around our addiction and causes us to form negative beliefs about ourselves: *I always fail. I'm not good enough. I'm not lovable. I don't deserve success.*

To help with my food addiction, Dr. Levy wanted me to enrol in a hospital program for eating disorders, either in a day program or as a six-week in-patient. On his advice, I applied for both programs and was accepted by both. This was what had created the conflict with Overeaters Anonymous. Whereas my OA sponsor had insisted on my total abstinence from binge-triggering foods, the two hospital programs allowed all foods in "normal" portions and required me to deal with my feelings before, during, and after eating. Both the OA and hospital programs insisted that I follow their rules and guidelines, and use their special tools for coping.

Deep down, I knew I couldn't — at least not yet — eat my trigger foods without bingeing, no matter how sincerely I worked on my feelings. My memories were too vivid of looking at a cake on a table, shaking so intensely for my sugar fix that I was like someone on heroin, unable to distinguish between the people around the table and that cake, because the people didn't exist for me as long as that cake was there. Though I decided that the hospital programs wouldn't work for me, neither would the conflict between my sponsor and my doctor, which is why I decided to leave Overeaters Anonymous to pursue a new path with Dr. Levy.

That path included taking pharmaceuticals. This was not an easy choice for me, but Dr. Levy helped me to understand that the compulsive path between my head and my addiction could never be shut down without this kind of intervention. I remembered how Zoloft had once normalized my life, and I decided to take his advice.

When Dr. Levy weighed me, I was only 118 pounds. He prescribed Concerta, which is a common treatment for ADHD, then told me that Concerta is also an appetite suppressant, so I should eat even if I wasn't hungry. He didn't want me to drink alcohol, and he told me that if I used recreational drugs of any kind that he would drop me as a patient. I had no problem skipping the alcohol and I no longer used recreational drugs, but I was confused about eating when I wasn't hungry, because I was trying to listen to my body.

Most recently, Vyvanse, an ADHD-approved drug that stimulates the central nervous system, has also been approved as a first-of-its-kind treatment for binge eating. Like all drugs, its use must be medically monitored for individual sensitivities and side effects.

Acknowledging that addictions arising out of ADHD require treatment involving brain chemistry could save many of you from needless suffering; however, I remain grateful to Overeaters Anonymous and other affirmative therapies for their role in helping me to create the purposeful life I always envisioned for myself.

Before moving on, I'd like to tell you about a guy named Scott Graham, whom I interviewed on my TV show, *Mind Matters*. As someone who speaks freely about having ADHD, he's an author, a camp counsellor, and a singer-songwriter who visits schools, teaching children that it's okay to have ADHD because it helps them to think outside the box.

I agree with him. I accept who I am, and now that I better understand myself, I wouldn't have it any other way. I know that when we ADHDers find something to be passionate about, our hyper-energy, our hyper-focus, our random daydreaming, and our willingness to take risks often lead to big accomplishments.

According to Dr. Russell Barkley, ADHD-friendly activities include athletics, the military, photography, acting, and all the other arts because they are fast-paced, creative, and conducive to independence.

Actors with ADHD include Jack Nicholson, Elvis Presley, Robin Williams, Will Smith, and Jim Carrey, who said he coped with his childhood difficulties by becoming the class clown. Even now, Carrey often finds it difficult to accept what others insist is "real" life. Similarly, Will Smith described his schoolboy self as the "fun one who had trouble paying attention." Though he struggles to read movie scripts, he has no trouble entering into the lives of the fictional characters that he plays.

Artists suspected of having ADHD include Salvador Dali, Pablo Picasso, and Vincent van Gogh, all noted for pushing the boundaries of art. Walt Disney turned his fascination with animation into an empire kick-started by the success of *Snow White*, despite his wife's prediction that no one would pay to see a full-length movie about dwarves.

Authors thought to have had ADHD include Charlotte and Emily Brontë, Mark Twain, Edgar Allan Poe, and Virginia Woolf — a trailblazer until the dark, depressive side of her condition led to her suicide. Child prodigy Wolfgang Amadeus Mozart wrote some of the world's most sublime music.

Given the obsessive training that goes into the creation of a sports superstar, it's not surprising that basketball great Michael Jordan was diagnosed with ADHD. So was Michael Phelps, the world's most decorated Olympian, with twenty-two medals. As a child unable to concentrate or sit still in class, Phelps was told by an exasperated teacher that he would never amount to much. That was before he learned to channel his formidable energy into swimming. He credits his ADHD for his success.[7]

Military figures thought to have ADHD include General George Patton; political ones, John F. Kennedy, both George W. and George H.W. Bush, Thomas Jefferson, and Abraham Lincoln; entrepreneurs include Andrew Carnegie, Henry Ford, William Randolph Hearst, Ted Turner, and Richard Branson, whose space-exploration company shoots for the stars.

Explorers like Christopher Columbus, who challenged our knowledge of the physical world, make the list of suspected ADHDers, along with Alexander Graham Bell and Thomas Edison, inventors who revolutionized our daily lives.

At the apex of this group of super-achievers are the world's two most famous scientists. Isaac Newton was a grumpy eccentric who became so engrossed in his physical experiments that he forgot to eat and who insisted on delivering his lectures to an empty classroom when no one turned up. Albert Einstein was slow to talk, obsessively repeated sentences, and became a forgetful adult prone to losing things. Yet, together, these two men invented the science by which we understand the laws of nature and chart the universe.

My mother used to tell me that if I could find something positive to put my passion and energy into, then I would feel much more fulfilled and successful. At the time this made me angry. I agreed with her, but I was frustrated because I felt stuck. I couldn't figure out a way to take the energy I was using to obsess over food and weight and put it toward something productive. It wasn't until I was finally diagnosed with ADHD and got treatment that I began to become unstuck. It took a lot of continuous effort to understand how to work with ADHD and to organize my thoughts. Finding the proper help and support was an important first step.

CHAPTER 5

A LANDMARK WEEKEND: SHOCK AND AWE

Though some people dismiss Landmark Education as a cult, I found the organization important to my recovery. Its programs, offered in twenty countries, are based on the techniques of est, a seminar training course founded by Werner H. Erhard. Because I was still reaching out for anything to speed my recovery, in 2007 I signed up for Landmark Forum, which is reputed to change lives.

The seminar, which cost five hundred dollars, took place on the top floor of a downtown Toronto office building. For three days, we would meet from 9:00 a.m. to 10:00 p.m. with breaks every few hours — 180 participants, all ages, all classes, all races. Anyone who decided by 11:00 a.m. of the first day that he or she couldn't handle the bluntness of the course was invited to leave with a full refund.

Despite my experience with Overeaters Anonymous, I was frightened by the thought of opening myself up to yet another group of strangers. At OA, we all suffered from some version of the same problem, but at Landmark I had no idea who anyone else was or what they were seeking.

Our Forum leader, David Ure, who we were told had already facilitated thousands of transformations, was an intimidating six foot five. In a deep, affirmative voice, he laid down the strict rules and principles by which we would be governed:

- Each of us must attend every session.
- No one could arrive late.
- Everyone who participated should expect to have many breakdowns and breakthroughs during the weekend.
- Our goal was to experience ourselves as satisfied and whole in the present moment, free from the baggage of our past.

During the program, we would be discussing ideas designed to stimulate us to review our lives and to share our insights. These would include the universal human desire to put on a good front for others; the "meaning" we project onto events that reflects our own values and expectations independent of the events themselves; and our tendency to defer legitimate pleasures to some indefinite future rather than live in the present.

Dealing with our "rackets" — our persistent resentments that give rise to fixed beliefs and habits — would be the focus of our self-exploration. Each of us would be asked to go into our rackets to create a story of our lives that would demonstrate some of our attitudes and behaviours. We were then supposed to get up in front of the group and spill our guts.

As person after person described how they had been beaten, raped, abandoned, injured in an accident, or traumatized by a loved one's death, I began to wonder what I had to talk about. Along with the speakers' pain, I heard a lot of blame — toward parents, toward partners, toward themselves. After each presentation, I listened as the Forum leader tore apart the storyteller's assumptions in a merciless dissection that was the psychological equivalent of neurosurgery.

I knew that if I didn't speak up during the Forum, I might never have the courage to reveal myself to myself, let alone to anyone else. Even so, I waited until the third day, though I knew I had to do it if I wanted to get anything out of the weekend. I could feel myself shaking uncontrollably as I bared my soul as a wife and mother, then admitted to my food addiction.

When I was finished, the leader bore down upon me with his large frame, dissecting and lacerating me with his powerful voice. He was mean and intense as he humiliated me simply by mirroring back what I had said.

He called me selfish and narcissistic, and what really hurt was that I knew everything he said was true. For ninety minutes, he performed this shock therapy on me in front of 180 witnesses. Much of the experience became a blur, because I began to lose consciousness in my attempts to tune him out. I know that I almost vomited.

When I was finally allowed to sit down, I was so confused I'm not sure what I was feeling. As I regained some composure, I saw that people were smiling at me as if they now knew and liked me. The veil of perfection revealing my pain-body had completely dropped from me for the first time in my life, and yet, strangely, it felt safe to be me.[8]

After the session, other participants sought me out to learn more about my story. They also thanked me for allowing them to access the hurt and hidden parts of themselves that my confession had brought into their consciousness. I could feel that others had been enthralled and transformed by what I'd said, and that it had made me popular for all the right reasons. I was no longer the perfectly turned-out woman who listened to everyone else without giving of herself. People seemed able to truly relate to me for the first time ever. I was experiencing, full force, the empathetic and compassionate side of others that I'd been blocking with my own projections and insecurities. Even though I wasn't sure what had happened during my ninety minutes of torture, I knew that I had experienced something wonderful from which there would be no turning back. I could also see how I had empowered everyone else in the room by being so open, just as they had empowered me through their confessions that reflected their own false biases.

The rest of the weekend was about creating a blank canvas on which I could design a new life for myself. My eating disorder had sidelined me into watching the game of life rather than fully participating in it, thus preventing me from enjoying my successes as well as learning from my failures. It had kept me small because I was afraid that being big would present me with bigger obstacles and more powerful challenges. I realized how deathly afraid I had been of people and their judgments. I also realized that everyone is, to some degree, afraid of everyone else. Once I navigated past that fear, I felt that nothing could stand in my way except my own lack of certainty about how to proceed and what my goals should be. I knew that learning and understanding how to communicate would be a big part of my future.

Throughout the Forum, we had been encouraged to contact those individuals in our lives with whom we had difficulty in order to make amends. I had heard so much about how people hated their fathers or their mothers or their partners that I remember feeling very blessed to have enjoyed such a close and amazing family. I phoned my mother to tell her how much I loved her and to apologize to her if she felt I had ever judged her or thought less of her because of issues involving my father. So many of my friends have told her that they wished she was *their* mother that I hoped she already knew all of this, but I still felt it important to put my own feelings into words. I also felt blessed to know that I had such wonderful sisters. We had always been so bonded, and my father was a part of that because he honoured and loved that unity among my mom, my sisters, and me.

At the end of the Forum, we were supposed to "declare our distinction," which meant creating a possibility for the future. I declared, "I've created the possibility of being present." I had never before felt fully present, certainly not in my body, but from that day forward, I *have* been present. Landmark was a turning point in ending my addiction and a pivotal point in my recovery for two reasons. First, it taught me to be present. Refusing to feed an addiction or use a substance and choosing instead to feel your feelings is a sure way to being present. Second, I created a powerful intention and held myself to it. Once you declare an intention to others, you have outwardly made that intention more powerful. The more people you share your intention with, the more you will hold yourself accountable.

On the Tuesday evening following the Forum, we participants were encouraged to invite others to learn about the program and to voluntarily register for an upcoming Landmark Forum. Of course, this type of soliciting is one of the reasons many people think of Landmark as a cult. Despite my awareness of this, I felt intrigued enough to volunteer to work in the Landmark office for a couple of months, phoning up potential customers to enrol them in a Forum. However, I know that while Landmark worked for me, it is definitely not for everyone.

At the Landmark office, I met another volunteer who told me about a telemarketing networking company that sold land line, cellphone, and Internet services. For every customer I signed up, I would receive a percentage of their telephone bill as commission, and when I signed up people under me, I would then receive a piece of their commission, and so forth down the line. I became so passionate about telemarketing that in four months I had two hundred people working under me. Not only was I on the phones, but I was also making presentations in people's homes. I loved it, and I was so brainwashed that I kept telling myself that I would soon be able to retire for life.

Eventually disillusionment set in, and I knew this wasn't for me; however, I did get an unexpected payoff that convinced me everyone should be a telemarketer for a while. I discovered that I was a great problem-solver and good at managing others as well as being a team player. That became an arrow pointing me to my niche in life, though it would take a couple of more years for me to understand that.

About the time that I quit telemarketing, I signed up for the Landmark Advanced Course, advertised as a way of turning personal intentions into public accomplishments. Though it was structured like the Forum, its effect on me was quite different, and quite unexpected.

My leader was Charlene Afremow — a seventy-eight-year-old woman with bigger balls than any man or woman I've ever met. She was a dynamo, and she terrified me so completely that I became frightened of my own shadow. No joke. I remember glimpsing my shadow as I washed my hands in the bathroom sink and jumping back two feet. I think that I must have dissociated. That's how tweaked I was. I felt picked on by the group, and too vulnerable to handle their judgment. I was afraid to get up from my chair. I was afraid to go home. When I built up my courage to ask Charlene why I was so frightened, she looked me in the eye and said, "You see yourself in me, and you're afraid of your own power. You remind me of myself at an earlier stage."

Since Charlene's comment didn't help at the time, I left the course feeling that I had received nothing from it, and afterward I was so depressed I spent four days in bed pulling myself together.

Naturally, I thought that would be the end of my Landmark experience. How wrong I was! A year later, in 2009, I received a call from the Landmark office inviting me to volunteer as a personal assistant to Charlene Afremow for a weekend workshop. *Charlene? The person who had traumatized me?* My initial response was, *No, never!* interspersed with a lot of expletives.

After I calmed down, I wondered if the universe was providing me with an opportunity to confront my fears to prove how groundless they were, and a conflicted dialogue launched in my head:

No, are you insane?
Yes, what else do you have to do that's as important as this?

Finally, I decided. Okay, how bad can it be now that I know what to expect?

When I entered the Landmark office, there she was — the old witch with balls! Charlene welcomed me as if nothing had ever passed between us.

My job was to look after all of Charlene's personal needs as her gofer so she could create a powerful, transformative weekend for those in her seminar. I was handed a list that spelled this out, with the most important items being: Buy food. Make and serve Charlene's meals exactly how and when she wants them.

Since I don't do anything halfway, I skipped the grocery store across the street to drive to where I could buy the freshest organic food, which I then prepared with love. Sometimes I went slightly over my budget, at my own expense, for edible flowers to put around Charlene's plate, because that's how I would want to be treated, and because I like to enjoy what I'm doing.

Charlene had arrived from California with a sore throat and a cough, and now here she was in a different time zone. Nevertheless this powerhouse woman conducted that whole weekend, from 10:00 a.m. to midnight, walking up and down, never sitting for second, not just teaching but catching people in mid-sentence, telling them what they needed to hear, as though she were hitting them with a ruler but without the ruler. Every two hours, to the minute, I had to serve her a concoction for her throat, and if I had ever missed doing so, I would have been in trouble. I still remember the recipe: one teaspoon of honey, one tablespoon of hot water, and one tablespoon of apple cider vinegar.

After only one day as Charlene's personal assistant, she and I had bonded so strongly that it felt like a love affair. Now, when I saw how others in her seminar feared her as I once had, I was able to explain to them how wonderful she really was. While she withdrew from those who shrank from her, she embraced those who confronted her. I watched this happen over and over, and saw myself even more deeply in those others, and I emerged from that weekend having made tremendous breakthroughs.

Charlene called me her angel, and afterward she let me spend the day with her, which was a privilege only a few ever experience with a Forum leader. I picked her up for lunch, then shared with her everything I'd felt about her in the past, and everything that was important about my life. She taught me even more about myself and especially about the need for perseverance. I *did* begin to see myself in her, as she had predicted, including my own power, though I still wasn't sure how to use it. She was like the Queen of Swords in the Tarot deck of cards — stern and sharp-tongued, with a keen intellect that cut straight to the point. I'm more like the Queen of Cups, intuitive and emotional, though I can be sharp-tongued as well.

I remember asking Charlene how she managed to teach the weekend's seminar with such dynamism despite her sore throat. She told me something I have never forgotten: "The way to deal with pain is just to be with it, to work with it and embrace it. Most people tense their bodies, then take a Tylenol in an attempt to shove it away, setting up a conflict so that it worsens and then keeps coming back."

When I pressed her about the source of her energy, she replied, with a mischievous smile, "I know what it's going to say on my casket — *Burnt Out.*"

Because I was receiving good value from my workshops, in 2010 I signed up for a Sterling Weekend for Women, which, like Landmark, advertised itself as intense, empowering, and transformational.

The Sterling Institute was founded in 1979 in Oakland, California, by Justin Sterling, a specialist in counselling high-powered women about the challenges of balancing their careers with their personal lives. His basic philosophy — that men and women are fundamentally different and that all life choices should respect that difference — resonated with me, because it was what my mother had taught me. However, his views have been severely criticized by those who feel he handicaps women in traditional ways, despite his insistence that he champions equality of opportunity and rewards.

To be accepted for the workshop, I had to be sponsored by a graduate willing to be my "big sister." Since the person who recommended the course to me *was* a graduate, this was no problem. At the initiating meeting, I declared that my goal was to learn to love and approve of myself 100 percent. I also wanted to deepen my friendships with other women.

Our weekend began with a nine-hour bus trip from Toronto, during which we were supposed to introduce ourselves to each other by declaring why we were taking this workshop. Our destination was Newburgh, a small town outside New York City, where we were booked in to a very basic hotel in the middle of nowhere.

As with Landmark, we were expected to share our deepest personal information with a roomful of over a hundred others, this time all women. One of Justin Sterling's key messages, as our group leader, was that we women usually underestimate our power. When one participant spoke regretfully about having left her husband after he cheated on her, Justin convinced her that she had the power to get him back from his current partner if she really wanted him.

Justin stated that men cheat because of their biology-driven desire for variety and the thrill of the chase, whereas women cheat because they feel their mates don't understand them. One of the greatest sources of gender discord arises from misunderstandings over the difference between long-term and short-term relationships. If a woman wants a long-term commitment from a man, she should signal this by not having sex with him for at least three months. Because women frequently fall in love with their sexual partners, they often suffer because of their attempts to turn short-term relationships into long-term ones, because this is usually impossible to do.

While I thought that Justin showed considerable insight into gender relations, I had trouble with his concept that *all* men and *all* women behave in these stereotypical ways.

As with Landmark, the Sterling weekend was conducted according to strict rules. Many of its big effects — or so I came to believe — were achieved through sleep deprivation. During one all-nighter, I remember walking through a corridor of women holding candles when I was too tired to see straight. In one exercise, conducted in the dark, Justin had all of us grieving until we sounded like a herd of cows mooing for our lost calves. I don't cry often, but because of all that loud emotion and heavy sadness, I began to cry, too, without even knowing why.

During the weekend, I both laughed and cried so much that my stomach felt as if I'd done five thousand sit-ups, and when the course was over, I had the greatest sense of relief, as if I'd been unburdened of a great weight I had been carrying.

As for what I learned about women — what I continue to learn — is how much pain we sometimes carry, and how hard we often are on ourselves and each other even though we're essentially all the same, with the same hurts and needs and strengths. Much of this behaviour stems from low self-esteem — it's practically an epidemic, colouring every aspect of our lives.

Programs like Landmark or Sterling are not right for everyone. But learning to overcome the assumptions you have about yourself, understanding how to be present, and overcoming self-esteem issues are important steps for anyone with an addiction.

CHAPTER 6

SEX AND SHAME: THE TANTRIC SOLUTION

My avoidance of sex was the result of shame connected to my over-eating. How could I feel turned on, playful, and joyful when I was used to experiencing my body as the hated battleground of my addiction and the unresolved insecurities of my childhood? I was especially anxious about the approach of summer, when I would be giving and attending pool parties. How could I face friends and acquaintances in my bikini when I still found it hard to face myself in the mirror? My father's long-ago critical voice was permanently lodged in my head: *Do you think Stacey still has time to become beautiful?* My mother's voice said: *Don't be a sex object. Don't encourage men to hit on you.*

Characteristically, the solution I chose to help me blast through my sexual inhibitions was an extreme one. In January 2010, I signed up for a course in tantric sex.

What is tantric sex?

Through research, I had discovered that it's an ancient religious ritual, dating from fifth-century India, in which intense and prolonged sexual orgasm is used as a channel to connect an individual with his or her spiritual self. While most religions treat sex as the enemy, Tantra utilizes sex as a sacred rite for surrendering the total self to the universal life force. It fires up the body's biological energy system as an expression of unity and love, not only for one's sexual partner but also for all things, seen and unseen.

The advertisement for the course that I chose promised to connect each participant to his or her sexuality, utilizing Eastern mind–body–spirit techniques suppressed for thousands of years. This would happen in a single weekend in a "safe, respectful" group environment, either with one's own partner or with a volunteer partner.

Twenty of us students and our female instructor gathered in a yoga studio decorated with Buddhist trappings. We ranged in age from twenty-five to fifty, and everyone seemed attractive, kind, open, and receptive.

The course was about exploring our five senses — touching, hearing, smelling, seeing, and tasting — in order to be present in our bodies during every moment of sexual activity. It was about staying out of our heads and focusing all of our intention on our *yoni* (female genitals) or *lingam* (male genitals) to produce an orgasmic rush of energy that would create a soul connection to a higher power.

I should state up front that, throughout the weekend, we never took off our clothes, engaged in sex, or touched our own genitals or anyone else's, but most of us did attain orgasms through group exercises and mind–body activities.

The average person might find the early stages of learning Tantra weird or slow or even boring. My own response echoed my first ho-hum experience of yoga. Since my expectations for yoga had been unfairly high, it took a number of classes before I understood the accumulative effect of its exercises, along with their underlying wisdom.

As in yoga, Tantra focuses on conscious breathing, since the breath is the part of ourselves that connects us to the rest of the universe. Some of our exercises, done either alone or with a partner, were about "feeling" our bodies' energy. For the first one, we vigorously rubbed our hands together, held them shoulder-width apart with palms facing, then very slowly drew them together, noticing the point at which our palms seemed to accelerate toward each other with a magnetic attraction. We also held hands in a circle, consciously feeling our collective energy swirl around the group. When we became fully present in our bodies, we focused our energy on our *yoni* or *lingam*, beginning to understand through their arousal that sex has everything to do with how confident we feel in our own sexuality. This meant each of us could have great "energy sex," including orgasm, with or without a partner.

To become sensuously present in every moment — hearing, seeing, tasting, touching, smelling — we used objects with different textures, like feathers, beads, and pearls, and different scented objects, like candles and incense. We walked outside, blindfolded, listening to birds, the sound of our footsteps, a passing car. We each took a raisin in our mouth and passionately made love to it for eight minutes — smashing it against our tongues, sucking it, experiencing the taste of passion. We stared into one another's eyes for long periods, then said something beautiful to our partner. We lay close together side by side on floor mats, then took turns rolling over all the others as a way of staying connected to our bodies — that was cool! We learned that masculine and feminine sexual cries are very animalistic and raw, but also very different, and we practised moaning and shrieking into each other's ears.

At the end of the weekend, we women dressed in sensual clothes — sarongs, bikinis, low-cut blouses, scarves. The men expressed their masculine sexuality by baring their chests and painting their faces. We nibbled on tantric foods, like tangerines and chocolate, reputed to be aphrodisiacs. We practised the sensuous, arousing exercises and breathing techniques that allowed us to bring our bodies to full awareness.

When we stood up to dance, I let myself throw off every constraint. My entire body moved like a crazed animal, and I became a wild, joyful lioness-diva. Given my sexual history, it took something to get that out of me in a roomful of people, but everyone else was dancing, too, moving the energies of their bodies down through their *yoni* or *lingam* in what Tantra calls a spiritual dance. We were having sex with our own energies, owning their thrilling power while staying present — something I had never imagined I could do. Finally, I dared to relax into full acceptance of my vulnerability, releasing so much repressed pain and so much wild pleasure, all of which allowed me to experience the uncontrolled power that had fuelled my food addiction. It scared me to think of what might have happened if I hadn't finally learned to channel this energy positively.

The whole weekend was a revelation. Who knew, given my history, that I would enjoy dressing up in sexy clothes, ditching all my inhibitions, and experiencing myself as a master lover in touch with the cosmos?

What did I take home from my tantric course that was permanent?

I came to understand that men love and respond to a woman who has the capacity to feel sexual within herself, since in pleasing herself she can more easily please her partner without having to think about it. This represented a big change for me, since I had always felt it was my partner's responsibility to turn me on, rather than knowing that the power to do so lay within me. My inability to experience orgasm had arisen from my fear of allowing myself to be vulnerable enough to surrender my body to pleasure, but now I knew that total vulnerability with my partner freed me sexually. When a woman is most relaxed, her hips are loose and her *yoni* is open to receive. Being tight in the hips cuts off movement and flow. I'd always had a hard time experiencing pleasure because I was working to give pleasure, not realizing that surrendering that role turned on my partner as well as myself.

Tantra taught me that sexual dynamism is all about owning my surging feelings of sensual arousal and release. It also taught me how powerful we women can be in our sexuality. When I was younger, this power felt dangerous, and then I lost it entirely when my eating disorder convinced me that I was never good enough.

Tantra brought out the inner child in me, allowing me to be playful and silly in the bedroom. There were times when I felt like I had left my body, forgetting where or who I was.

Tantra helped me to understand the role that ADHD had been playing in my sex life: keeping up a constant, conflicting chatter in my head; preventing me from experiencing and enjoying the needs, desires, and pleasures of my body; blocking me from touching ecstasy.

I came to understand that sex can be either slow and gentle or animalistic, and that I was eager for both. Because men come quickly to the boil, they need to slow down both for themselves and for their partners. Learning how to breathe properly is very important for sustaining an erection, and since many men don't fully understand women's bodies, we need to teach them that we must be warmed up first. Our bodies are our sanctuaries, our possession, and their prize, and if they want that prize, they must understand how to win it.

I learned that orgasm isn't the ultimate goal of sex but rather the spiritual pathway to a deeper union with the self, your partner, and the universe.

I came to understand that just by staring into another person's eyes, you can lose yourself so completely that it's like physically making love, or maybe even deeper and more intimate because such a connection is about your soul, your partner's soul, and the collective soul.

Along with all these lofty possibilities, I'm also realistic. While worshipping your mate may guarantee full love and acceptance in the bedroom, living with your partner on a daily basis can cause resentments to build up alongside different goals and agendas, making it hard to hold on to what begins to seem like a distant fantasy. Sometimes, it's also legitimate to want, to need, and to ask for more space.

CHAPTER 7

TRANSFORMATION: BECOMING REAL

started seeing my therapist in 2006, and saw her for ninety minutes each week for many years while recovering. She is non-judgmental, smart, spiritual yet logical, trustworthy, well-balanced, patient, and compassionate. When I see her now, I always trust that she has my best interests objectively in mind. I find talking to her useful, especially when I am going through a period of crisis or making an important decision.[9]

Over the years, my therapist has given me the ability to communicate the feelings and thoughts that I used to repress. She's done this by assuring me that everything that goes on in my mind is normal. When I realized, through talking everything out, that I had no reason for shame or uncertainty, I began to see that anything I considered negative would pass, allowing me to count my blessings.

My therapist is the person who taught me, through example, more about how to be a therapist than anything I learned in college. When seeing my clients, I try to adopt her way of being.

When she first attempted to explain the theories of Carl Jung, one of the founders of psychoanalysis, she might as well have been speaking Chinese, I was that clueless. It took hours of listening to words — like *shadow* and *persona* — that I considered jargon before I began to understand not only what they meant but their connection to me.

According to Jung, the human psyche consists of many parts, of which I will talk about three — the ego (the conscious self), the persona (the mask we show to the world), and the shadow (our repressed side, which contains the parts of ourselves, both dark and light, we don't want to own).

In *The Strange Case of Dr. Jekyll and Mr. Hyde*, Robert Louis Stevenson provides a literary example of Jung's theory of personality. While Dr. Henry Jekyll is experimenting in his laboratory, he discovers a potion that unleashes the shadow side of his personality — the conscienceless and murderous Edward Hyde. Gradually, Hyde overwhelms Jekyll, despite the struggle of the well-intentioned part of Jekyll (his ego) to keep the peace, and this results in the death of the whole personality by suicide.

In Oscar Wilde's *The Picture of Dorian Gray*, a young man makes a deal with the devil in which his portrait (his shadow) ages and turns ugly as a result of his conscienceless, debauched lifestyle while his physical self (his persona) remains ever youthful and handsome. In both Mary Shelley's *Frankenstein* and Bram Stoker's *Dracula*, the shadow side of the scientist and the count, in the form of a monster and a vampire respectively, break free in a rampage of evil that overwhelms and destroys the rest of both men's personalities.

One of the goals of therapy is to integrate the shadow rather than allowing it to remain hidden. When repressed, the shadow becomes dominant as the negative part of ourselves that we unknowingly project onto the rest of the world. On the simplest level, this means recognizing, becoming responsible for, and dealing with the petty emotions that mar our daily lives and lead to quarrels, regrets, and frustrations. When all parts of our personality are in balance, we experience ourselves as whole, productive, and free, which allows us to take credit for, and to enjoy, our accomplishments and pleasures.

What Jung calls the shadow isn't all "evil" like Mr. Hyde. It's only when its content remains hidden, unknown, and uncontrolled that it creates unhappiness for us and others. When we make our shadow conscious, we release its energy and even its wisdom, which we can then put to good purpose.

As I came to understand, my shadow was my eating disorder — the chaotic and depressed part of me that I wanted to hide because it was too frightening and too deeply rooted in pain. My persona was the upbeat self and skinny body that I was always trying to perfect. My ego was the belea-guered "me" who struggled to keep peace between the person I pretended to be (my persona) and the creature I feared I was (my shadow).

As long as I failed to face and understand the contents of my shadow, it remained outside my control — the part of me that I projected onto friends and family as envy, anger, resentment, and blame for my own shortcomings.

Why did my shadow cause me to binge on chocolate cake when I didn't enjoy it after the first couple of bites? What was I really hungry for that made the cake seem like a good substitute? What was missing in my life that I wanted so badly? Why was my appearance so important to me, and why did I need to hurt myself so much because of it?

As the first-born in my family and an only child for five years, I had an exaggerated need to make my parents proud, especially my father, by becoming "perfect" in his eyes. As a perpetual people-pleaser, I lost track not only of who I was but also of my own legitimate needs. While polishing my outer shell (my persona), I neglected my inner development. At the same time, I internalized other people's criticisms of me, real or imagined, as part of my shadow, so that I became my own most severe and constant critic.

What was I hungry for? As I came to understand it after decades of failed diets, jobs, and friendships: a self of my own and a life filled with meaning. It was my shadow's pitiful voice, crying out for fulfillment, that I tried to shut up by stuffing its throat with food. By refusing to leave me in peace, it forced me to learn who I was, which unleashed my desire to lead a purposeful life. That was the wisdom of my shadow.

Another part of Jungian theory that at first confused me was the "anima" and "animus," which my therapist described as the masculine and feminine sides of each one of us. When interpreted through this lens, the stories of *Sleeping Beauty* or *Cinderella* aren't about young women rescued by men. They're about the feminine side of a personality (nurturing and loving) embracing the masculine side of the personality (the desire for achievement and adventure) to create a fully realized self.

This helped to explain the confusion I often felt between my "girlie" side, which I pampered and indulged, and my strong drive to be something more than a wife and a mother. This was the hard-nosed part of me that refused to settle for being less than I could be, and that launched me on a relentless journey of self-discovery. This was the part of myself — my animus — that was still without the kind of goals and achievements that would make me feel complete as a person.

When my therapist suggested in 2006 that I keep track of my dreams, I dutifully did as I was told, but considered it rather pointless. After I discovered the significant role dreams could play in understanding myself, I compiled about one thousand pages of them, including their interpretations.

To Jung, dreams are like nightly letters from the unconscious self to the waking self, and provide us with information vital to our psychic health and happiness. An important clue in interpreting any dream is how it makes you, as the dreamer, feel — anxious? depressed? optimistic? hopeful? Another vital clue is the knowledge that each figure in a dream can express some part of you, the dreamer. To unlock a dream's meaning, it is also very useful to have some knowledge of dream symbols so as to understand how each symbol reflects what is happening in your life.

When I dreamt about helping an elderly great-aunt push her wheelchair through obstacles to safety, my therapist reminded me that I was both the great-aunt in need of help (against my crippling addiction) and the person able to rescue her. The fact that my great-aunt was, in real life, a Holocaust survivor, indicated that I, too, was a survivor.

In our daily lives we usually communicate with words, but in dreams we communicate with images. It's the use of this "other language" that makes our dreams difficult to translate until we become familiar with the new vocabulary. What better way to convey both powerlessness and survival than through the image of a wheelchair-bound elderly woman who escaped the Holocaust?

While many dream images come from our own lives, some are universal. People across all cultures are afraid of the dark because of what it might hide; therefore, darkness in dreams symbolizes things that are frightening because they are unknown and hidden.

The scariest parts of fairy tales often take place in dark forests. Little Red Riding Hood must escape a wolf; Hansel and Gretel, a witch. By defeating the wolf and the witch respectively in their collective unconscious, they emerge from the darkness, transformed from frightened children into confident youths en route to adulthood.

When I told my therapist about a sad dream in which I stole a white narcissus, she told me a Greek myth about a beautiful youth named Narcissus. When Narcissus saw his reflection in the water, he fell in love with it, not understanding that it was his own image. Then, when his reflection didn't return his love, Narcissus tumbled into the water in grief and drowned. After his corpse was laid on a funeral pyre it disappeared, and only a flower — a white narcissus — was left. This myth gave rise to the psychological term *narcissist*, meaning a person obsessed with the self.

Though I consciously knew nothing about Narcissus, according to Jung, our unconscious self has direct access to the "collective unconscious," which contains the accumulated wisdom of the human race. What better way to warn me about the danger of my obsession with my appearance than the poignant myth of Narcissus in love with his own reflection?

Jung believed that events that happen to us in dreams are equal in emotional power and reality to those that happen to us in our waking lives. I sometimes have vivid dreams in which I make amends to people with whom I've been in conflict. This releases pent-up anger, guilt, resentment, and remorse, and creates the healing that is sometimes unavailable in ordinary life because of lack of opportunity.

Today, I can say with certainty that my dreams helped me to understand not only who I was but also who I would become.

My therapist introduced me to Sandplay, another technique based on Jungian principles that uses symbol to access the unconscious.

The first time I walked into her office, I was startled to find her surrounded by hundreds of miniature figurines — princesses, witches, dragons, snakes, cats, dogs, horses, rabbits, castles, cars, houses, et cetera. As part of my therapy, she invited me to choose a bunch of these miniatures and arrange them any way I chose in one of two sand trays filled with wet and dry sand, respectively.

I like working with symbols, and I believe I have an intuitive talent for doing so. Even in everyday life, if, for example, my watch stops, I take it as a sign that I need to be more mindful of time, perhaps to slow down or to move forward more quickly, depending on what's happening in my life. If I lost my passport, I would see that as having to do with my identity; if my house keys, I'd wonder why I didn't want to go inside my house.

I view astrology in the same way. Though I don't live my life according to any chart, I find that astrological symbols and their meaning provoke me into thinking more deeply, and keep me more aware and conscious. Many people don't understand this, or shy away from it because it's hard work, but if I don't pay attention, the universe is likely to hit me harder on the head with something I can't ignore, like maybe an accident or an illness that brings my life to a standstill.

Though I'm describing my therapy as if I were an all-knowing observer, that's not the way I lived it. During the early years, I was still struggling to understand my shadow in order to free myself. I felt grateful that Neil, my husband at the time, hung in with me through countless ups and downs, providing strength, goodwill, and grounding.

I remember one evening, on the way home from a big dinner, when I wanted Neil to stop at a store so I could buy some ice cream.

He told me, "You're not allowed ice cream."

I insisted. "Take me to the store."

As we drove around the parking lot, he begged me, "Please don't do this. Call your OA sponsor."

Since the car was moving very slowly, I opened the door and jumped out. I bought ice cream, peanut butter, and chocolate sauce, plus four pieces of my favourite chocolate, which I ate immediately — I couldn't get it into my mouth fast enough.

When I returned to the car, Neil was disappointed and angry with me, which increased my desire to eat. Then, when we arrived home, we had an argument over the kids, which I used to further justify my bingeing. After Neil went to bed, I devoured the ice cream and peanut butter.

All during dinner that evening, I had felt that Neil was deliberately irritating me. Maybe he was and maybe he wasn't. When you're an addict, your judgment can't be trusted, but — on the other hand — you're not always wrong. Those close to you try to support and protect you, but sometimes they also play into your problem, using it as an excuse for their own negative behaviour. It's hard, when you're always questioning yourself, to sort this out.

Being a mother is also a continuous and amazing learning experience. I grew up wanting kids, and I can't imagine life without them. I'm close to both of my wonderful sons, and I believe I'm a good mother, but recognizing and meeting their individual needs and challenges was especially difficult while I was dealing with my own issues. The older was seven and the younger three when I got a grip on my addiction. That was in 2007, when I was thirty-two. They both know that I had an eating problem, but now they see that I eat a balanced and mostly healthy diet without obsessively restricting anything. I knew I had to stop myself before I negatively impacted their lives. And destroyed my own.

After decades of struggle, I discovered that the only thing harder than getting better is being sick, which is something we addicts don't understand until we *are* better. Therapy meant remaking the values of a lifetime. It was often tough going, but now, when I read over my journal entries, I can barely remember who that damaged person was. It was difficult for me to learn how to trust my body enough to know when it was hungry and when it was full, to surrender my fears related to my weight, and to accept my feelings instead of stuffing them down my throat by bingeing. Eventually, I came to believe the little shadow-voice deep in my core that warned me, If you don't do something meaningful with your energy, you are going to lose everything. Just like Narcissus did.

Programs like Overeaters Anonymous taught me to be grateful for what I have instead of yearning for what I don't need, to be a seeker who never gives up, to visualize the future that I want, and to trust the universe to guide me to that future.

I didn't want to hide in my shadow anymore. I wanted the insanity to stop so I could be of service to the world by offering it my light. Though I didn't yet know how this was going to happen, or where this would take me, I was so determined that I believed I couldn't fail. I understood, finally, that the way I'd been living didn't work, and that I had to surrender "my way." By surrendering, I accepted that addiction is a part of my life and that my addiction had been in control of me. When I surrendered, I accepted that I needed to gain control. I had to stop fighting against myself and move toward acceptance.

Make no mistake: My shadow didn't give up its power over the rest of me overnight, and the support I needed didn't just happen to come my way. I had to want it enough to create it for myself. As an addict, if you invest only 50 percent, you'll be lucky if you get even that much back. I found no shortcuts or quick fixes, but what I learned has stayed with me. New knowledge and new experience can't be taken away because they become a part of you. I would not be who I am today without having gone through what I did, and since I now know, like, and love myself, that realization has transformed my "lost years" into a blessing rather than a waste.

Yes, I'm happy to confirm that by the end of 2007 I was binge-free. I remember so vividly when seven days without bingeing seemed a triumph. Now it has been years. As a bonus, my weight has stabilized at around 120 pounds, which I used to consider my skinniest — that number is just a guesstimate, since I don't weigh myself any more.

I no longer fear food. I can have the cakes or cookies or carbohydrates I once feared and walk away after just one bite. This took many years of practice. It took many failures to get to where I am today. Many times throughout my recovery I questioned myself. I had a hard time being confident in my choices about food and exercise. But now I no longer deal with my feelings by stuffing food down my throat, so there is no need for me to use or abuse my body by bingeing or restricting. When I look back, I realize it had nothing to do with the food and everything to do with the feelings I was stuffing down.

An important footnote: While I'm markedly different than I was in 2007, I'm still unabashedly the same person at my core, which is partly what this next part of my story reflects.

The thing I most wanted as a reward to celebrate my new sense of self was not a birthday cake or a gallon of my favourite chocolate ice cream. What the girlie side of me wanted was plastic surgery to restore my breasts to what they had been before I ruined them with extreme nursing and pumping. Not to look like Pamela Anderson or Dolly Parton — just like Stacey Gorlicky as she had been "before" rather than "after."

When I broached the subject with my mentors, I was still bingeing some of the time, and both Dr. Levy and my therapist urged me to wait before making this kind of decision. A year later, the desire still hadn't gone away. Though my therapist is an entirely natural person, I believe she felt better about my determination to have the augmentation surgery when I began to dream in an intense and happy way about having already had the procedure and being thrilled with the result.

I underwent the operation in the fall of 2007. At first I loved the result, just as in my dreams. However, after a while I began to brood that I should have chosen a bigger size. Soon I was comparing my breasts to other women's and feeling sad because I knew my chest would shrink as the swelling from the surgery went down. When I told my therapist about my anxieties, she urged me to surrender to my present reality, to accept myself as I was, and to understand that I was fully a woman before the operation as well as now.

While still worrying about what I would say to my plastic surgeon at our next appointment, I called my ex-sponsor from OA, knowing that she would be as blunt as necessary. I was right. She told me that I was obsessing over my breasts the way I used to obsess over my weight, and that if I had another breast enlargement, I would soon find something else about my body that needed fixing, until I became a plastic-surgery junkie who looked like a clown.

Nasty, but it was the jolt I needed.

All the wisdom I had absorbed from my mentors and all my experience as an ex-addict clicked in. I remembered my *aha* moment at the mall, when every cell of my being assured me that I *did* love myself as "good enough." I remembered to be grateful for all that I already had, and I vowed that the thing that filled the space in my life left by emotional eating would not be another addiction.

CHAPTER 8

READY FOR LIFTOFF:
SEVERE STORMS AHEAD

At age thirty-four, I felt secure enough to become excited about what my life could be like without my eating disorder. I knew it would have to be something BIG to fill the void left by my addiction — something I could pursue with the same passion with which I'd once tracked down and devoured chocolate sundaes. Yes, the future looked hopeful, but also daunting.

The careers I had tried — gift-shop co-owner, makeup artist, real estate agent, network marketer — had never satisfied me, and my mediocre academic record seemed to bar me from higher aspirations. I wanted to be taken seriously while doing something that would excite my easily bored, wandering ADHD mind.

I put this message out to the universe with a new intensity, praying for doors to open, because if you ask for nothing, that's what you get — nothing. I begged, I pleaded that someone or something somewhere would hear my prayers. Essentially, I was back to repeating Steps 11 and 12 from Overeaters Anonymous.

Step 11: I will seek through prayer and meditation to improve my conscious contact with God, as I understand this higher power, praying only for knowledge of God's will for me, along with the power to carry this out.

Step 12: I will practise these principles in all of my affairs because being of service is the greatest gift I can give to myself and another human being.

I didn't have a clue what I was praying for — certainly, as a child, I'd never said, "Mommy, I want to be a psychotherapist."

Gradually, I began to attract people who guided me in the right direction. When I told a therapist I'd met at the Sterling weekend that I'd love to do what she was doing, she told me about Toronto's Transformational Arts College of Spiritual and Holistic Training (TAC). "They offer professional courses for becoming a therapist."

"But how can I possibly catch up?"

"You don't need credentials beyond secondary school. You just have to be willing and able to handle the tough, intense work."

I immediately contacted the school, and in September 2010 enrolled in their full-time, one-year Spiritual Psychotherapy Training course. It was exactly what I wanted — a combination of holistic and spiritual practice with more traditional psychological methods.

In the past, I'd quit every career I'd started because my eating disorder had stolen my energy and my brainpower, but I was no longer that person. I was on a steep learning curve, but loving every second of the challenge. Oh, I had my doubters, especially my husband and my dad: "There goes Stacey again, obsessing about psychology the way she used to obsess about food. You'll quit, as always. You're wasting time and money."

I replied to both of them, "How could I ever quit this? I'm thirsty for it; I'm hungry for it. I can't ever get enough of this because now I'm feeding my soul."

I really didn't care what anyone said to discourage me because I knew that I'd finally found my purpose after years of searching.

In September 2011, I graduated from Spiritual Psychotherapy, along with courses in Discovering Total Self and Spiritual Direction, which included grief counselling. After that, I studied addiction counselling at McMaster University.

Despite being hit by three life-changing traumas within three months at the end of 2011, I still graduated with honours from my Spiritual Psychotherapy course.

These traumas were:

1. My sixty-year-old father was diagnosed with lymphoma.
2. I struck a five-year-old boy while driving an SUV.
3. I was thrown from a galloping horse, broke a rib, tore the skin off my back, sustained a concussion, and damaged my hip, neck, and spine through whiplash (which resulted in minor retrograde amnesia).

First, my father's cancer. For forty-two years, he'd been waking up every morning at four to start smoking the first of three packs of cigarettes. Despite the urgent pleading of my mother, my sisters, and me, he swore he would never quit.

Suddenly my father did quit, cold turkey, the way I once quit marijuana. He'd been feeling feverish, and I guess he suspected something might be wrong with him. A week later, he was diagnosed with cancer.

He was in shock, and as we were a close family, so were the rest of us. But we were also convinced he would survive, and we came together like the Care Bears to make sure that happened. We joined our hearts and showered him with enough love to overwhelm his own doubts and fears.

What Dad had was Hodgkin's lymphoma, which is possible to recover from, so we kept telling him that it was an easy form of cancer to beat, even though there's no such thing.

He required many needles, which he hated, and then he had to endure chemotherapy. One of us always drove him to the hospital and stayed with him throughout the treatment. On one occasion I had to leave him at home alone afterward so I could go to school, since class attendance was compulsory if I wanted to graduate. When I arrived back, he'd been in so much pain that he hadn't moved from the couch where I'd left him. He hadn't even pulled a cover over himself.

My mother always says, "You're born alone, and you die alone, and no one else ever truly understands your pain, no matter how close you are."

After watching my father go through six months of cancer treatment, I came to believe that was true. Now, when my clients tell me no one understands their suffering, I think of my father's struggle with lymphoma, and me with my eating disorder, and I know they're more right than wrong.

Despite Dad's extreme pain, he never once took a morphine pill. I didn't understand that until a friend who'd been through something similar told me, "Patients like your father believe, consciously or unconsciously, that by taking morphine they are signalling that they are ready to die. Your father's way of fighting is to keep aware of his world and in touch with his own feelings through every step of his journey. For him, that's the right decision. For other cancer patients, relieving their pain just makes sense."

During my father's illness, I felt blessed to be taking my TAC grief-counselling course on conscious dying. This course, conducted by John Pollard, who also teaches at York University, helps connect people to their higher selves and to the universe during and after a crisis. It taught me how to be present with my dad, even in the most ordinary of circumstances. While driving him to pick up my son from school, we'd listen to the birds, see the blueness of the sky, feel the sunlight, and enjoy the most phenomenal moments of shared awareness.

My father, as my friend suggested, wasn't ready to die. Before cancer, he'd lived in the past and in the future, seldom in the moment, and too often he was angry and unreasonable, though he has a good heart. I believe he experienced a rebirth, because with cancer, part of you actually does die before you go into recovery. Coming through all that was like winning the lottery. My father became softer, more relaxed, more grateful. He even began to pay attention to some of the healing music I played for him, instead of closing that door. He also lost a lot of weight, and now he's able to keep it off because the muffins and the Blizzards aren't as important any more. When he and I sit side by side for a meal, I think we both understand on some wordless level that food always represented love to us, but now it's a nurturing bond rather than a toxic one.

My dad's life has shifted in a positive way, and after seeing how completely my mother was present for him while he was ill, he has become more thoughtful to her, in ways like running her bath water. He always loved her, but now you can see that he cherishes her.

Through my father's cancer scare, our family learned not only how precious life is, but also the need to treasure every moment.

My second trauma took place while my father was still struggling with cancer. It was a Wednesday, which was my longest day at TAC because I was taking an extra course in the evening. During a ninety-minute break, I went for dinner with a friend, with the intention of also stopping at the Indigo bookstore on Yonge Street. It was 6:00 p.m. on a beautiful October day, still light out without a cloud in the sky, and I wasn't speeding. No cars were coming as I turned off Yonge onto a street with a parking lot across from a Mastermind toy store. That's when a little child seemed to fall from the sky.

I heard a terrible thud as my SUV hit him so hard he went all the way under the car to the other side. My passenger shouted, "You hit a kid! You hit a kid!"

I was in shock. "Oh my God, oh my God!" I gasped. As I climbed out of the car, a doctor who'd witnessed the accident ran to help the child.

Now the child's mother was screaming, "Who hit my kid?"

I told her, "I did. I'm so sorry. I have a five-year-old boy, too." I hugged her. "I don't know how this happened. I don't know what to say."

By then, an ambulance, a fire truck, and a police car had arrived — someone must have called 911. The boy was conscious and crying, which was a good sign. Witnesses were coming forward to reassure me, saying "I saw what happened. He ran out of nowhere. It wasn't your fault."

All the witnesses were on my side, which surprised me, since a child was lying on the street and I wasn't soliciting support. As I later figured out, he had been so excited when he saw Mastermind, with all those toys, that he ran from his mother's grasp.

After the boy was put on a stretcher, I phoned Neil. Can you imagine receiving a call like that from your wife? *I just hit a kid.* I was shaking so hard, I had trouble describing what had happened, let alone believing it. Now Neil was also in shock.

The police questioned me, and after an hour and a half, I was free to go. The boy was fine, except for a mild concussion. *Fine? How could that be, with his blood all over the front of my car?*

When I arrived home, the first person I told was my five-year-old son — I probably shouldn't have, but he was the one most on my mind, and he's a strong little guy.

Though I wasn't charged, the accident wasn't over for me. I kept having flashbacks — in my sleep, during meals, during conversations, and certainly while driving. I kept replaying the whole scene from the instant I began to turn my car to park — the ghastly thump, the screaming, the blood, the sirens, the stretcher, the mother, the police, the witnesses.

My condition wasn't hard to diagnose: post-traumatic stress disorder.

Fortunately, my psychotherapy training also told me what to do. I did a couple of sessions of eye movement desensitization and reprocessing — a therapy utilizing lights, designed to heal trauma by releasing the memories from the part of the brain where they have become isolated and obsessive.

I wanted to get in touch with the child's family to assure myself that he was all right, and to give him some of the toys that had caused him to run toward Mastermind; however, the police refused to allow me to make contact for what they described as legal reasons.

This heart-stopping experience, like my father's cancer, once again underlined for me the preciousness of life, along with the vulnerability of each one of us, not just from day to day, but from moment to moment.

My own accident occurred during our family's Christmas vacation on the Caribbean island of St. Maarten. Two days before we were due home, we were all becoming rather cranky from being cramped in a small space — just one of those low times during a vacation when everyone is supposed to be having fun. Since I thought it would be a good idea for parents and kids to have a brief break from each other, Neil and I took the unusual step of leaving the boys with the hotel's babysitting service so we could go horseback riding.

We were riding together as a group, when suddenly my horse decided to gallop. We were at the top of a steep mountain, and he just bolted down as if spooked. Horses are sensitive to energy, and this one — his name was Freddy — must have felt my backlog of frustration. Freddy probably wanted me to get the hell off his back so he could return to the stable. I was wearing jeans and a pair of flip-flops — *What was I thinking?* We flew by rocks, we flew by trees, we flew by cacti, with me gripping the horse so hard with my legs that I burned through my jeans. I knew I was going to be thrown, but I didn't know just when. My life actually did flash before my eyes, and next thing I knew, I was down.

Up I jumped. This was instinctive, despite my being in shock. Probably I needed to prove to myself that I hadn't snapped my spine.

By the time Neil and the others caught up, they saw that I was standing and decided I must be okay. They walked me down to a safety station, where my back, with its skin ripped off, was disinfected with peroxide, which made me scream.

I knew that something was terribly wrong, but I listened as the others reassured me that I was fine.

Later I phoned my mother, who said, "You need to go to a hospital. You could be bleeding from the brain. People dismiss these accidents and two days later they're dead."

Neil took me to a doctor even though he insisted my mother was overreacting. I was given OxyContin for pain relief.

The next day, the kids wanted to go to the beach. The trip to the beach took over an hour, during which I was delirious with pain, despite the codeine that I was now also taking. Every part of my body still seemed to be hurting.

Once I was in the ocean, the waves were so big they sucked me under and whipped off my sunglasses. I became hysterical, accusing the universe of treating me unfairly. *Why are you doing this to me? First, my dad has cancer, then I strike a kid, and now my body is broken. Why have you taken away my rose-coloured glasses when I need them so badly? What do you want me to see more clearly?*

Of all those catastrophes, the one that seemed most important at this moment was the loss of my four-hundred-dollar sunglasses. I strode up and down the beach, trying to find my glasses, staring at people, convinced someone must have stolen them, and shouting at everyone and anyone to help me find them.

I couldn't settle. But now I know that the experience of losing those glasses was superficial compared to everything else I was going through. I didn't have the energy, strength, or patience to deal with those around me who told me that I was fine after the fall. I wasn't listening to my own needs and my own body — two very important things that many of us overlook in recovery.

Fortunately we were going home the next day. Once back at the hotel, all I wanted was to get to a Toronto hospital for a full body scan. My Toronto doctors diagnosed a broken rib, a severed breastbone, a concussion, whiplash, and torqued hips, as well as the obvious back abrasions where my skin had been torn off.

I was still obliged to attend TAC classes if I wanted to graduate, since if I missed even one, I would have to make it up the following year. I was taking Percocet for the pain and going to a chiropractor and an acupuncturist to enable me to sit through classes because nothing — nothing! — was going to prevent me from achieving my degree. I also used my TAC knowledge to connect mindfully with my "inner body," which meant travelling emotionally into the parts that were hurting — my neck, my hips, my ribs — to ask why each was in pain and what I could do about it. Though this may sound crazy to some people, the emotional, physical, and spiritual effect of this practice can be profound.

What my body told me was that I had been too harsh with it through bingeing, starving, and over-exercising. What it needed was for me to just "be" with it, to breathe into it, to meditate, to be kind to it, to be still. To understand that less is more.

When I did that, I began to experience the most amazing energy, along with life-changing insights. This felt like the out-of-body, near-death experiences so many people describe, in which I was suddenly able to view my life from a higher perspective. I became aware that I had been trying to take energy from others instead of finding it within myself.

I began to see that so many of my anxieties were petty and unworthy of my present stage of development — like those missing sunglasses. I also began to see which people no longer belonged in my life because I no longer felt safe with them, or because we had developed different needs and different values. Once again, this reinforced, in a deeper, more intense, more personal way, what I had experienced through my father's cancer and the car accident: that I must cherish and make the most of every single moment.

Afterward, I felt so different — so much more conscious — that I went around asking friends and family, "What was I like before my accident?"

Most agreed that I seemed to have changed. Even Neil, who didn't understand a lot of my stuff, asked, "Where did Stacey go?"

The physical healing itself was slow. For example, during yoga, my hips felt locked for a long time, and I still have scar tissue on my left side where I had a very bad bruise.

No sane person chooses trauma as a form of learning, but the combination of those three fateful months, with their three near-fatal events, my training courses, and my experience with addiction turned me into a psychotherapist. I was ready to live my dream of helping others to transform themselves. What I did not yet realize was how much personal change also lay in wait for me just up the road.

As I've said many times in this book, all of us are on a journey, whether we realize it or not. When you consciously choose to make that journey a dynamic one, with greater self-awareness as a goal, then change is what you get. Your expectations, your values, your motivations change, and what worked in the past may no longer work in the present or feel right for the future.

Neil and I separated in May 2014. That summer, I began to date a man who worked in the same field as I do. His name is Mark, and we share the same passion and purpose through our careers and profession: to treat mental health problems, addiction, and trauma with an integrated program of neuropsychology and cutting-edge mind–body techniques. Mark and I arrived at this same place of commitment to others through our own addictions. Our connection was strong and immediate.

I moved in with Mark in March 2015 while my divorce was in progress, and that June, I merged my therapeutic practice with his.

Divorce is never easy for children, but I believe that, paradoxically, I have become closer to my sons, Tyler, fourteen, and Kyle, ten. I feel more present with each of them because I am happier. Though still kids, they are growing up into affectionate, well-behaved, smart, and sensitive young men, and I'm proud of the way they have matured.

Today, when I am going through a crisis or a rough time, I know that food will not make me feel better. I feel the pain of my situation rather then stuff food down my throat. Bingeing does not allow me to work through my issues; it only puts everything else on pause.

I have made a full recovery; there are no slips or thoughts of bingeing. If I do have a moment when I think, "I'm fat," it passes quickly. I don't obsess over it. I remind myself that I am not a machine that needs to be perfect all the time and that I need to be gentle with myself. Understanding how to deal with my feelings, as I was forced to during those difficult periods, was an important step in my recovery.

Life is good.

PART III

PAYING IT FORWARD

Knowing your own darkness is the best method for dealing with the darkness of other people.

— Carl Jung

CHAPTER 9

LIES WE TELL OURSELVES: TEARING UP THE OLD SCRIPT

When a client enters my office, the first thing I want to know is what he or she hopes to achieve through therapy. Is she here of her own volition? Was it a crisis that brought her to this decision? Did someone close to her present her with an ultimatum? Is her therapy court-mandated?

Next, I want to know if my client has a specific issue, like addiction, or if the problem is more general, like depression. What experiences, good or bad, has this person had with therapy in the past? How long does he expect to be in treatment, and how often is he able to attend?

In asking these questions, what I'm looking for are basic indicators of therapeutic success: honesty, a desire for treatment, a willingness to take risks by venturing into the unknown, and the client's level of personal insight.

It's a cliché of therapy, but one worth acknowledging, that emotional problems, especially those related to addiction, typically begin in childhood.

By the time we start school, most of us have already created a story about who we are, based on the attitudes and values of our families, and how well our own emotional and physical needs have been met. Contributing factors include how many siblings we have and where we are in the family birth order; which sibling we believe to be a parent's favourite; our family's economic circumstances; family traumas; and the state of everyone's health, especially our own.

The stories we create around our identities as children are a major factor in how we conduct our daily lives as adults — the critical choices we make, how we interact with others in ways both good and self-destructive, and the happiness we allow ourselves. If we're very lucky in our upbringing, the stories we invent will be loving and supportive, and will encourage us to develop to our full potential. Most often, however, what we absorb is a mixed bag of positive and negative influences that reflect where our parents were in their life's journey as well as cultural pressures and accidental circumstances.

We have many positive experiences as children, but often a single negative experience will stand out the most. The negative event will stay with us and override positive experiences. This is believed to be because negative emotions like fear and sadness trigger increased activity in a part of the brain linked to memories. For example, you could have had many great and positive experiences in relation to your body, but the one time that your parent or friend at school called you fat stayed with you. So that one negative comment increased activity in the part of your brain related to memory and created a trauma. In turn, because this memory is so powerful, it has led you to believe this to be true about yourself, creating your own reality.

As we get older and live with this reality, we look for events to reinforce it. We create a self-fulfilling prophecy by doing things that reinforce what we already believe about ourselves, whether true or not. What ends up happening is that we create a "feedback loop." It may begin with the negative thought, "I'll always be fat." So you make the effort to diet. However, if your method is to binge, which leads to overeating, your weight will likely just yo-yo. What has happened is that your actions have led to the embodiment of the original thought, which finally leads to the outcome you originally imagined. This negative outcome will feed the negative initial thought and strengthen it, as you will now feel like you have undeniable proof of failure. The more this happens, the stronger the negative initial thought will become. Working through the trauma of past wounds and negative beliefs is the only way to move through distorted beliefs that we carry with us.

Since people seek out therapists because they are troubled, my role often involves helping a client rewrite a sad and pessimistic life story into a positive, realistic, and inspiring one. It's then that the old script can be torn up instead of continuing to function as a self-fulfilling prophecy.

A little girl who has an unstable, abusive, toxic, or non-existent relationship with her father is likely to develop into a woman with a negative view of her appearance, leading to a deliberate attempt to make herself unattractive through poor grooming, obesity, and ill-fitting and unisex clothing. Her lack of self-esteem is often acted out through fear of or disdain for all men, coupled with a hunger for affection. Alternatively, she may exaggerate her sexuality through provocative dress, leading to promiscuity based on a hunger for male attention. Both of these types of women are likely to be attracted to unavailable, unsuitable men who will hurt and abandon them. They will have problems with physical and emotional intimacy even in a good marriage, and will regard all criticism, however well-intentioned, as a personal attack.

Girls who have an unstable, abusive, toxic or non-existent relationship with their mothers often have the same issues as those with a poor relationship with their fathers; however, they are more likely to blame other women for their unhappiness. This leads to jealousy and over-competitiveness, often beginning with their female siblings. They may identify with men and have few, if any, female friends. As parents, they may be either neglectful or smothering while remaining emotionally attached to their own critical mothers in a futile attempt to gain their approval.

Men who have an unstable, toxic, or non-existent relationship with their fathers often have trouble understanding how a man should act. If their father is abusive, they may become abusive to women while being overly attached to and defensive of their mothers. Since they lack a role model, they are likely to abandon their children, or to compensate by making good fathering a cherished goal.

Men with a dysfunctional or non-existent relationship with their mothers may become adults who distrust all women, who look for a woman like their mothers from whom they can squeeze love, or who expect their partners to fill their emotional void. If that void remains unfilled, they will keep seeking replacements in the belief that the problem is the current woman, not themselves.

Any of these destructive patterns, derived from a negative relationship with a parent, can result in addiction. If either parent is an addict, the stakes are dramatically higher.

Tina was an attractive, forty-five-year-old woman with a beautiful smile. As someone who was extremely loving and nurturing, all she wanted from life was happiness for her two children, whom she'd had with different fathers. It was only when Tina's obesity began to interfere with her ability to care for her children that she panicked: *What is the point of living if I can't nurture my children? Would they be better off if I were dead?* Tina's low self-esteem also caused her to search for love by serving as the long-suffering caregiver of her difficult mother and the unreliable men in her life.

Tina's father had abandoned his family when Tina and her twin brother were five. When they were ten, the family was involved in a car accident in which her brother was killed, while she and her mother sustained only minor injuries. Though her mother was suspected of having fallen asleep at the wheel because she was exhausted from working extra shifts as a waitress, she was never charged.

After the accident, Tina's mother became a weekend boozer, and when she was drunk, she was mean to Tina. Tina sensed that her mother blamed her for surviving while her brother had died. Tina, too, blamed herself. She and her brother had always fought to sit in the front seat. Despite the fact that it was Tina's turn on the day of the accident, she had let her brother have that privilege for reasons she could never explain.

Because of her father's departure, Tina grew up believing that men would always abandon her. Because of the circumstances of her brother's death, she internalized the idea that any misfortune to anyone close to her would always be her fault. Overeating was her way of feeding her guilt about her brother. It also served to make her unattractive to men and thus protected her from further abandonment. Since her mother's constant criticism caused her to fear women, she had few friends, and blamed "sexy vampires" for breaking up her two marriages.

Who could be happy living out a script like Tina's?

———————————

Once a client understands the roots of her story, creating a more positive one is challenging but doable. I love the saying "It's simple but not easy." Because Tina's children were her motivation for getting well, I had to convince her that taking care of herself was the first step in looking after them. For pleasers like Tina, it's wise to repeat the instruction that aircrews always give their passengers: Put on your own oxygen mask before trying to protect your children.

Tina's first task in overcoming her food addiction was dealing with her false and burdensome sense of blame. For early-family work, I often employ "inner-child" therapy. This means guiding a client on an inward journey in which she meets, and has a conversation with, her child-self. Afterward, the client describes to me what the adult thinks of the child and what the child thinks of the adult. Eventually, the adult understands that the child she has been blaming had no control over the traumas in her family's life. Realizing this usually leads to the release of deeply repressed pain, too dangerous for the unprotected, vulnerable child to express at the time of the events. In Tina's case, she was as much a victim of her father's abandonment as her mother was, and as innocent of her brother's death as her brother himself.

I was able to make the innocence of Tina's child-self clear to her by asking whether she blamed her children for their fathers' abandonment. I also asked her if she blamed her oldest child for the broken arm that her youngest child had sustained while they were both chasing the family dog. Even the thought of this horrified super-protective Tina and made it easier for her to rescue her own child-self from the blame she had projected upon her.

Since Tina's mother perpetuated these beliefs, it was important for Tina to either deal with her mother on an adult level of self-protection and forgiveness or to consider abandoning the relationship as toxic. Given her mother's level of self-damage, a relationship based on mutual self-awareness was not possible. As a nurturer, Tina chose forgiveness. By now, she was strong enough to see that it was her mother's own unbearable guilt over the accident that had caused her to shift blame onto Tina and then drown herself in alcohol.

False beliefs are most lethal when they remain unconscious, because they can then result in irrational and self-punishing behaviour. Recognizing this is not only the key to getting better but also prevents us from hurting others. We do not want to hurt our children, our friends, our lovers; however, we are all wounded individuals who learn that pain seems easier to carry if we transfer the burden to someone else. But this just causes it to accumulate. I have never met a mother who intentionally wanted to hurt her child, but that's what Tina's mother did, because she did not understand how to deal with her own suffering.

By rescuing herself from her mother's projections and her own false beliefs, Tina opened herself up to healthier relationships. She now understands that it was not just bad luck that caused her to marry two men who would abandon her and their children. She also understands that forgiving her mother involves establishing boundaries against her mother's unchecked verbal abuse.

Though Tina is still working to curb her overeating, now it's more a practical matter of correcting bad food habits rather than dealing with an addiction fed by a perpetual supply of loneliness, anxiety, guilt, and shame.

In Tina's new script, she is an honourable, lovable woman quite capable of taking care of herself and her children. She has made friends with a female colleague whom she once envied, and hopes someday to trust herself enough to find a man worthy of sharing her life.

For clients like Tina, who have unfinished emotional business rooted in the past, revisiting the wounded child-self and allowing both the child and the adult to experience the pain connected to that trauma allows them to move forward. For all of us, it's wise to remember that no matter who or how successful we are, each of us has a "Little" inside who constantly affects our "Big" in both positive and negative ways. While it's our Little who is most vulnerable to hurt, it's also our Little whose mischievous spirit allows us to laugh at silly things, to enjoy playing with a kitten, and to delight in finding exactly the right colour of paint for the bedroom. Healing our Little also encourages our Big to extend tolerance, compassion, and friendship to others.

Some clients have no patience with the idea of exploring the past to heal the present. Instead, they enter therapy with specific problems they want solved in the here and now. Edward was one of these, though in many ways his problems echoed Tina's. He came to me because of obesity brought on by binge eating and because of relationship problems with his girlfriend, Melanie.

At thirty-eight, Edward claimed that all he wanted was to be a good father to his two children from two previous marriages. He had not wanted another woman in his life, but Melanie, a beautiful twenty-five-year-old model, was very enticing. At the same time that he worried about how he could hold on to her, he worried even more about how to handle an anorexic cocaine addict who sometimes paid for her fixes by working as a high-class prostitute.

As Edward talked about his woes, it became apparent that his fatal attraction to Melanie was based in how much she needed *him*. This had also been true of Edward's two ex-wives, both of whom had been addicts.

Whenever Edward was without his kids or Melanie, his angry "monster" came out, causing him to binge and then to throw up. Bulimia was especially shameful to him because he saw it as a female behaviour. Though Edward had been bingeing and purging from a very early age, he dismissed his childhood as "normal."

For clients like Edward, I often use cognitive behavioural therapy (CBT) to correct the thoughts and values that produce negative outcomes in adult life. The more obsessive and fixed these false beliefs, the more they will invade every aspect of a person's present life, and the more stubbornly he or she will fight to prove that these beliefs are true and normal.

In Edward's view, he was a compassionate, good guy of whom women took advantage. His first wife — a sex addict — ended up marrying one of her lovers. Though he supported his second wife, an alcoholic, through a successful rehab, she left him to devote herself to her career as an interior designer. He'd been these women's rescuer, their confidant, their backbone, their all-weather guy, whom they'd used and then dumped, hurting him so badly he was now emotionally unavailable to himself and to others. The quality Edward most hated in women was ingratitude — and these women had taken advantage of him, which made him feel anger and self-pity.

Since I'm a big fan of journaling as a form of grounding, I suggested that Edward keep a record of the ordinary events in his life and his feelings about them — the quarrels, the petty annoyances, and the disappointments, as well as the events that made him happy. Though Edward was reluctant, he eventually came to count on this process of "letting off steam" as an important part of his day. On the surface, his entries often appeared innocuous, but a deeper look revealed that Edward carried over to his workplace the fixed and distorted beliefs that upset his personal life.

Edward was an accountant at a financial institution, where his most pressing current problem was his relationship with his boss, Barbara. When she had joined the company five years earlier, Edward had mentored her in their complex work environment. After Edward's former boss retired, Edward had expected to be promoted to the management position. Instead, Barbara had been given the job. Edward was incensed. Once again, he was the dupe of an ungrateful, manipulative female. He had been Barbara's white knight, teaching her everything he knew, and now look what had happened — trickery and betrayal!

Since Barbara's character was unknown to me, I had no way of assessing how justified Edward's anger against his former protégé was. However, reading between the lines of Edward's journal revealed that he often took time off work for personal problems, frequently arrived late, and failed to meet deadlines. When questioned, he admitted that in the past he had often expected Barbara to cover for him. The relationship, in short, had not been as one-sided as Edward chose to believe, nor his entitlement to promotion so clear-cut.

Not surprisingly, Edward blamed his bingeing on the turmoil created by the women in his life. Any one lapse usually resulted in a week of all-out gorging. He was especially fond of anything caramel, served with large helpings of self-pity.

Events in Edward's life that should have been happy fell victim to his distorted all-or-nothing thinking. Edward had a beautiful tenor voice, but when he was cast as the understudy to the lead in a community-staged opera, he interpreted this as yet another failure, even though he would have almost as many chances to perform as the lead. It was only because he was beginning to understand his self-defeating patterns that he hung in rather than quit. Months later, when his recovery was even further underway, he was thrilled to perform onstage, with his children and one of his ex-wives in the audience.

As with Tina, Edward's bingeing became less of an issue as he gained more confidence. His biggest struggle remained Melanie and all that she represented in his life. As we discussed their relationship, Edward gradually opened up about his childhood.

Edward's mother had been sexually abused by her father, for which she blamed men in general, including Edward and his father. When she was drunk, she would beat up Edward, and if he brought friends home, she would shame him with insults about his weight and his clumsy behaviour, even though she was the one blindly stumbling into walls. When she disappeared for days at a time, Edward was torn between fear that she would never return and fear that she would. When she reappeared, she was sometimes drunk and disorderly, but sometimes affectionate and energetic enough to prepare delicious meals. These brief flashes of happiness convinced Edward that his mother really loved him despite her behaviour.

Edward's father was a passive man who always treated his wife with respect. Because he didn't know how to deal with the anxiety of raising Edward and his sister, he may have had a few affairs as a coping mechanism. Edward alternated between feeling sympathy for his father and contempt for him as a loser.

Edward's mother eventually overdosed while away on one of her binges — an event for which both Edward and his father blamed themselves.

This was the family Edward had dismissed as "normal."

The only relationship that Edward had known was as a codependent.[10] Without a woman like Melanie in his life, he didn't have any identity. As a kid, he clung to the idea that his mother loved him because it was too heartbreaking and scary to admit to himself how alone and vulnerable he was. When the women he tried to rescue as an adult left him, he had to believe the problem was their ingratitude, not the fact that he felt he was unlovable. In his desperate efforts to rescue others in pain, what he really yearned for was someone to rescue him.

Once Edward began expressing himself in his journal, and then to me, he was finally able to open up to his father. Eventually, the two established a gentle relationship based on their mutual love of Edward's children. Edward also made tenuous peace with his boss, Barbara, based on his realization that he had never wanted the management position in the first place. He still fails to acknowledge that the underlying pattern in his relationship with Barbara might be the same as that with his wives. Instead, he seizes on the main difference: "Barbara wasn't an addict!"

Edward is still struggling with his feelings for Melanie and working on his food addiction.

Twenty-three-year-old Darryl came to see me because she was confused about her sexual identity. Because she sought sex with both male and female partners, she wanted me to answer for her the question "Am I a lesbian or am I straight?"

Darryl enjoyed the fact that men were physically bigger and stronger than she was, which made her feel feminine and vulnerable. But at the same time, she feared male power. She would describe sex with men this way: "The cock is piercing and passionate and feels so good, but it's also so scary."

Darryl also liked to describe how much women turned her on. She loved watching lesbian porn. She also loved the fact that her female partners were soft and delicate with her, caressing her body as if they cared about her. Drawn to women who were more beautiful than she was, she yearned for those who were unattainable yet felt sad with the desirable ones she attracted because she felt she didn't measure up.

Darryl found it difficult to say no to any man who wanted sex because she felt that saying yes was the only way to gain a man's attention. When she was bored, there were a few she could call on to hang out, smoke a joint, and have sex. Afterward, she would be angry at herself for following the sexual path society imposed on her instead of being true to her desire for women. Contradicting herself once again, she said she wanted to marry a man someday and have kids to please her parents and to feel "normal."

Though Darryl seemed unashamed of either her desire for sex or her willingness to act out her fantasies, the four to six hours a day she spent watching lesbian porn was creating a guilt issue for her. As with so many of my clients, Darryl also experienced shame over her body, which, at five foot three and 130 pounds, she considered too fat. Though she assured me her food issues were under control, she often complained about overeating. In fact, during our sessions, Darryl talked as much about food as she did about sex. Though she was desperate for compliments, she found them difficult to accept. She even questioned why she had been given a boy's name, for which she had been teased in school, and which she blamed for making it even more difficult for her to figure out her sexuality.

After Darryl and I discussed her childhood, her body-image issues and confusion about her sexual identity began to make sense.

At age ten, Darryl was sent to Toronto's Hospital for Sick Children because she was anorexic. During six months as an in-patient, she was fed what she remembers as enormous amounts of food. After her release, her parents continued to monitor her food intake so strenuously that she lost the ability to choose for herself.

Darryl's mother, Lana, was a beautiful and skinny woman who didn't have to worry about what she ate. Having a mother like Lana was difficult for Darryl, since she believed her stylish mother would be repelled by having a fat daughter. As the family's breadwinner, Lana had an executive position at a Fortune 500 company, while Darryl's father, Bruce, was the angry and resentful family caretaker. He looked after Darryl and her younger brother, Lance, while occasionally supplementing the family income with odd jobs.

Darryl described Bruce as a control freak with a "raging" personality. He would thrust his face into hers, screaming that she wasn't going to amount to anything. He would also vent his anger by whipping her with a belt or with his hand, usually while Lana was at work. If this happened while Lana was at home, she would try to protect Darryl. At the same time, she would make excuses for Bruce: "He's just stressed out. You need to be more respectful of him."

During our sessions, Darryl would repeatedly ask me the question that began our therapy: "Am I a lesbian?"

I would reply, "That's something you'll have to answer for yourself."

She would then express her confusion by saying, "How can I be a lesbian when I love sex with men so much?"

Eventually I told her, "You're asking the wrong question. What you should be asking is, 'Why am I so unsatisfied, no matter whom I have sex with?'"

I suggested that Darryl keep a journal in which she explored her feel-ings about sex — not just about the encounters she was already having, but about what, ideally, she would like to feel while in the arms of her partner, what needs she was seeking to fulfill, and how she wished to feel about herself after sex.

Through her journaling and our conversations, Darryl came to under-stand that her bisexual partnering was an attempt to find the emotional support she had failed to get from either of her parents — the father who beat her and the mother who didn't love her enough to protect her. When Darryl was with a man, she feared his strength and potential control, just as she feared her father's domination. When she was with a woman, she felt physically but not emotionally safe, because she could not live up to her mother as a role model. Unable to find her own sexual identity, Darryl went back and forth between male and female partners, feeling as lost and con-fused as she had as a child. She was yearning, reaching out, but not receiving. She also came to understand how she was self-sabotaging. Whenever she found big, safe male arms to fall into, she would push that man away. At the same time, she was afraid of her vulnerability in female commitment and that her lesbianism would be regarded as blasphemous by her family.

Despite the energy Darryl was putting into sex, the only thing her meaningless relationships did in this futile attempt to fill the void inside herself was numb her feelings.

Eventually, Darryl found herself ready to attempt to answer the ques-tion, Am I a lesbian?

In Darryl's parents' marriage, the stereotypical male/female roles had been reversed. Her mother was the breadwinner. Her father was the care-taker, albeit one who beat her up. To add to her confusion, her brother, Lance, was gay but high-achieving like her mother. Though his sexuality was accepted in the family, Darryl did not see how she could be an under-achieving lesbian and still find self-worth.

Of her own volition, Darryl stopped watching the female porn to which she had become addicted, finally understanding that sex with a woman was never going to heal her relationship with her mother. She also came to realize that the biggest barrier to her establishing a loving partnership with a man was her rage against her father's violence and control. As a child, she did not have a voice big enough to speak up to him during his fits. As an adult, she came to understand that his taunt "You're never going to amount to anything" was a projection of how he saw himself and had nothing to do with her. She made it clear to him that if they were going to have any kind of a meaningful relationship, he could no longer yell at her or raise his hand to her. Though Darryl said that establishing these boundaries was the scariest thing she had ever done, once she released her voice, she found she was more than a match for her father's fake power.

As we continue to play out unfinished stories and to heal wounds from our childhood, sooner or later we realize that as conscious beings we are drawn to compensate for what was missing in our past. Darryl is currently hoping to find a man who is sweet and soft but who understands and respects his masculine side. Though her father never modelled this possibility for her, she no longer believes that all men are bullies.

It's the rare person who reaches adulthood without developing "cognitive distortions" that are either mildly or wildly debilitating. We are all born innocently receptive to the influences around us. If we don't understand why we are being punished, we may develop a sense of injustice that festers as resentment or causes us to lash out in anger, and results in even more punishment. Alternatively, because we love and fear Mommy and Daddy, we may decide they are always right. That means we must be to blame for being punished, and if that keeps happening to us, then we must be bad. If we are bad, we may feel perpetually guilty and ashamed, or we may decide deliberately to be bad in order to draw attention and punishment to ourselves.

All of these decisions, made moment by moment, are based on too little information and minimal experience. As children, we don't really know why Mommy and Daddy act the way they do, so we invent a story that makes sense to us. We create an identity from the bits and pieces we have glued together out of our vulnerability and ignorance. Then we spend the rest of our lives demonstrating to others who we believe ourselves to be or — if we don't like ourselves — hiding who we believe ourselves to be. Much of the time, we don't know the difference.

Dr. Aaron T. Beck, one of the developers of cognitive behavioural therapy, has isolated some of the common cognitive distortions that trap us in negative loops:

All-or-nothing thinking: Why did I bother with all that training just to come in a lousy second-best?

Overgeneralization: Since I always have a terrible time when I go anywhere by myself, it's better to stay home.

Filtering out the good: It would have been a great party if only I hadn't spilled eggnog on my blouse.

Mind-reading: If he thinks treating me at an expensive restaurant means I'll have sex with him, he's got cement for brains.

Fortune-telling: I know she'll end up dumping me, so why bother?

Minimization and magnification: It was only dumb luck that got me this interview, and if I don't get this job, I'll never get another in my field.

Cynicism: Why should I believe you when you say you like my painting? What's in it for you?

Rigidity with rules: If everyone stayed away the way she does because her kid is sick, we'd have an empty office.

Mislabelling: Why would any guy want a fat person like me?

Blaming: Okay, so maybe I had a couple too many, but she was the one who wanted to go to that club.

Always being right: I told him that if we got a dog, that would be the end of our garden. Why doesn't he ever listen to common sense?

I find CBT an easy therapy to use with my clients because I once possessed so many distorted views about myself. Now I employ CBT to treat a wide range of disorders, including addiction, depression, phobia, and anxiety. The aim is to create greater flexibility in a client's thinking, which leads to the exercise of greater flexibility in choice and action.

As an exercise, why not go over Dr. Beck's list, item by item, and see how many of your own habitual attitudes you can discover? Take your time and don't get hung up on the specific examples suggested in the list — be free-ranging as you apply each distortion to your own behaviour. If you can't break through your own defences, look for the attitudes typically displayed by people you know or by my client Edward. At least it's a start.

This exercise is especially useful for times when you find yourself obsessing over some fresh disappointment or hurt. If you're in familiar territory, ask yourself, Why does this keep happening to me? Write out the incident from your own point of view, then try to see the assumptions underlying your hurt or disappointment: *Why am I always defending myself? Why do people pick on me? Why am I always blamed for telling the truth?* After you vent your own feelings, try seeing the incident from the other person's point of view. Try to be as passionate in expressing his or her feelings as you were with your own. Now, reassess the total situation as objectively as you can.

If you catch yourself in a distortion, try an affirmation that corrects your attitude. For example, if you are a blamer: *I accept responsibility for my own thoughts and actions.* If you're always right: *I respect the views of others just as I respect my own.* For a general affirmation: *I love and accept myself.*

Choose a sentence that's simple and easy to say. Repeat this positive message whenever a negative message is present in your mind. Say it as many times as you can throughout the day, even if you don't yet believe it to be true. Say it to yourself as you drive or work out or have a shower. Envision and own it until it enters every brain cell so completely that you radiate it to others.

Positive affirmations are one of the simplest and most effective ways to lighten your mood on any day, and even to change the false beliefs of a lifetime. Transformation can be simple, or it can be complicated.

CHAPTER 10

ANOREXIA:
DANCING WITH DEATH

Anorexia shares many characteristics with overeating: a distorted body image; a hatred of the body leading to a hatred of the self; a need for perfection; fear of food; vomiting and purging; avoidance of, or obsession with, weight scales and mirrors. All of these things create guilt, anxiety, and shame.

Because I'm a therapist specializing in eating disorders, every year a few anorexics make their way to my office, often brought there by their worried parents.

When I met twenty-one-year-old Dorothy, she weighed only seventy pounds, her cheeks were concave, and her complexion was bluish. She admitted that she had a problem, and was very scared and shy, but she stated up front that she didn't want to do anything about it. It was as if she nursed the impossible hope that I could make her healthy while allowing her to disintegrate.

When I asked Dorothy what she ate in a day, she replied, "A handful of carrots and a handful of grapes — at most."

If she ever ate more, she felt obsessively guilty. "I don't deserve to eat. I just want to be skinny."

Dorothy never came back to see me after the initial appointment because the idea of change was too scary for her. I wrote to her, worried about her safety, urging her to seek help, but she wasn't ready to face her tragic reality.

———————

While overeating can lead to death from side effects like diabetes, heart disease, and other maladies, for anorexics the route from *diet* to *die* is far more direct. According to Dr. Blake Woodside, medical director of the Eating Disorder Program at the Toronto General Hospital, about 10 to 15 percent of anorexics will die from their illness, and another 10 to 15 percent will become chronically ill.

"Anorexia nervosa is primarily a young woman's illness, too often treated by therapists with traditional methods that are successful for other mental illnesses, but not for this one," says Dr. Woodside. "A discriminatory attitude develops that such patients are untreatable, which is far from the truth. The therapeutic route may be complicated; it may be long; it may even be something we can't explain or describe easily, but the good news is that 60 to 65 percent who seek treatment will make a full recovery so they're eating normally and are okay with their body's weight and shape. Five years later, they can say, 'My illness feels like a bad dream, like something that never happened. I don't know how I got that way, and I will never ever go back there.'"

I learned about Naomi through a phone call from her father, who told me that his twenty-year-old daughter had an eating disorder and needed to talk to someone. Whenever a parent contacts me, I always try to ascertain whether the child is willing to make changes because forcing someone into recovery never works. Though he assured me that Naomi was ready, her defeatist attitude during our first appointment did not suggest a good prognosis.

At five foot nine and weighing only ninety pounds, Naomi had already spent six weeks in hospital being treated for anorexia. After she had gained thirty pounds, she was dismissed, with no attempt to help her to understand her mental illness or its severity. As soon as Naomi returned home, she determinedly tried to lose the weight she had gained. She didn't think she had an eating disorder, and she hated her "fat," cumbersome body.

Naomi had dropped twenty-five pounds of her hospital weight when I received her father's phone call. She told me that she felt fine, that she had plenty of energy, and that she knew from having already seen other therapists that this treatment wouldn't work. She justified her attitude by saying that her last therapist had admitted she could do nothing for Naomi and had terminated the treatment.

Though I did my best to help and support Naomi, she seemed thinner at every appointment. She was losing her hair, her skin was dry, her speech was slow, and her mind was impaired so that she had difficulty comprehending the therapy necessary for her improvement. The only reason she seemed to hang on to life was because of her love for her sister, who sometimes drove her to appointments and then waited for her. The sister would plead with Naomi to eat enough to gain weight, but nothing anyone said seemed to get through to her.

I knew that Naomi needed to be readmitted to hospital as soon as possible. With her permission, I contacted her GP about her case. Before any action could be taken, Naomi passed out at a mall where she was shopping with her mother. An ambulance was called, and Naomi was resuscitated after losing consciousness for quite a few minutes.

This experience shocked Naomi into realizing she had a problem. She also knew that if she didn't voluntarily admit herself to a hospital for recovery her GP would commit her to a psych ward as a danger to herself.

Fortunately, Naomi had a concerned family who could afford private care, so she didn't have to go on a long waiting list — a wait that perhaps would have resulted in her death. Instead, she spent the next six months — a far longer treatment time than for most in-patients — at a California recovery centre that specializes in eating disorders. As her recovery therapist told me, the critical shift for Naomi came the day she started to sing. The sound of her liberated voice brought her back to her own life, so that she began living for herself instead of for her sister.

After Naomi returned home, we again started working together. As before, her main wish was to lose the extra weight she had put on at the clinic. This signalled to me that we had a critically short time-frame in which to assure her survival. Though she was terrified about opening up to me, I found her sufficiently improved to do the intense work necessary for a full recovery.

When Naomi was very young, her father and brother often made disparaging comments about women's bodies. While Naomi and her sister were not fat, they felt they could never measure up to the ideal image of how they *should* look. Even at seventy pounds, Naomi had hated her "fat" thighs and stomach, and usually thought she was the biggest person in any room. Not only was Naomi frightened of being called fat, but she was also frightened of being merely "average." She was convinced that men liked perfect women, the skinnier the better. Achieving such a body became an obsession with her, even though that kind of perfection doesn't exist.

Naomi experienced much shame over her disorder and also had major trust issues with men. Boundaries were a big problem for her, so she would often have sex with partners because they wanted it — even if she didn't — and she didn't know how to say no. She thought pleasing men would cause them to stick around, but the opposite proved true, so she was always being hurt by rejection.

Because Naomi couldn't control others — *who can?* — she insisted on controlling her body. Her eating disorder also drew the attention she craved as someone "special." Anorexia felt like a safe and familiar hiding place, even though it was a dangerous disease that was killing her. Like Dorothy, she felt worthless — like someone who did not deserve to nourish her body in order to live. The very thought of eating — or of even looking at food — was difficult for her.

Persuading Naomi to unlock her feelings was difficult, but Jung's concept of the shadow helped her to understand that her anorexia had turned her into a shadow of herself, and that this shadow had taken over her life. Fortunately, her experience in the California recovery centre had also taught her that her shadow liked to sing, the way she used to as a child. Joining a community choir helped Naomi embrace her shadow in a big step toward discovering that life was worthwhile. Singing required her to "tune up" her body, which meant accepting food as a necessity. It also gave her a healthy way to earn attention rather than getting it through her disorder. Though it was a struggle for Naomi to learn to feel hunger and to associate it with the need to eat, she gradually built that bridge. Her new-found confidence also helped her to set boundaries in her relationships with men.

It was truly amazing to share Naomi's journey, and to help her not only to survive but to begin to thrive.

Why did Naomi fall victim to anorexia, while her sister, with a similar family background, did not? For one thing, despite having the same parents, Naomi and her sister didn't necessarily inherit the same risk factors.

Also, according to Dr. Woodside, a person's vulnerability results from a mixture of inherited and cultural factors. "Think about genetics loading the gun and the environment pulling the trigger. If you have the genes for anorexia or bulimia, and you live in a society like the Fujian Islands, where people don't diet, you're never going to activate your genetic risk factors. However, if you live in a society like ours, with a lot of dieting, then you may do so. Most people who diet just gain weight — I mean, that's the most common result of dieting for the population as a whole — but if you have the wrong genes, and something negative happens to you, and you try to diet it away — which is societally approved behaviour — you can activate your liability."

The incidence of death by starvation has risen sharply over the past few decades. In today's skinny-loving Western world, it's very easy for a woman with low self-esteem to slide down that slippery slope. Even someone of normal weight has only to lose a few pounds to be showered with compliments. How confident, how svelte, how sexy she feels in her size-four, form-fitting clothes, perhaps with a stylish new hairstyle, too!

In the fifties, the voluptuous hourglass figure of Marilyn Monroe was the definition of sexy desirability. By the sixties, stick-thin supermodel "Twiggy" (Lesley Hornby), with her moon face and big eyes layered in false lashes, established the waif look. In the mid-nineties, Calvin Klein turned Kate Moss — emaciated, androgynous, with pale skin, protruding bones, and gaunt, dark-circled eyes — into the poster girl for heroin chic. Though this "graveyard look" created a backlash, thin is definitely still in. In a 2007 survey of models by the British Fashion Council, 50 percent believed that anorexia and bulimia were significant problems in their industry, and 70 percent confirmed the trend toward thinner models.

As British actress-model Elizabeth Hurley famously remarked in 2005, "I'd kill myself if I was as fat as Marilyn Monroe!" Monroe's measurements, taken from her studio clothes, revealed that she had a 35-inch bust, 22-inch waist, and 35-inch hips. At five foot five, her weight fluctuated between 115 and 120 pounds — nothing to be ashamed of!

In 1983, the shocking death of thirty-two-year-old singer Karen Carpenter did for anorexia nervosa what Rock Hudson's death would do for AIDs two years later: brought it into public awareness. Karen — half of the brother-sister balladeer duo The Carpenters — was a wholesome girl next door in contrast to the increasingly wild rockers dominating the music scene. Her pointless death was made especially poignant by one of the Grammy-winning duo's biggest hits, "We've Only Just Begun."

The nineties ushered in other high-profile deaths from anorexia: American gymnast Christy Henrich in 1994, age twenty-two, and American ballerina Heidi Guenther in 1997, also age twenty-two. In 2006, Uruguayan fashion model Luisel Ramos died at age twenty-two; her sister Eliana, also a fashion model, died less than a year later at just eighteen. Israeli model Hila Elmaliach also died in 2007, at age thirty-three, after struggling with anorexia for twenty years. French model Isabelle Caro died in 2010 at age twenty-eight. Before her death, she allowed herself to be interviewed and photographed with her spine protruding through her taut skin, as a dire warning to others. At her thinnest, Caro weighed only fifty-five pounds, which were stretched over her five-foot-five frame.

In industries like modelling, where anorexia is perceived to have career advantages, those most at risk are too often pushed to the brink by agents and coaches. The article "The Most Infuriating Thing You Will Ever Read About the Modeling Industry," published on April 22, 2013, in the online magazine *Slate*, revealed just how low vultures will swoop in their desire to live off the bones of young anorexics. As Katy Waldman reports, caretakers at Sweden's 1,700-bed Stockholm Center for Eating Disorders had to change their patients' outdoor routines because modelling scouts were stalking critically ill young women and offering them a chance to become living coat hangers for their agencies. One even attempted to recruit a girl so emaciated she was confined to a wheelchair!

For those suffering from an eating disorder, every aspect of their lives is affected, especially when that disorder is anorexia. While experts agree that it is a complex disease that arises from multiple causes, one cause is overwhelmingly linked to this condition. As verified by Dr. Woodside, 60 percent of his anorexic patients have been sexually or physically abused.

It's not hard to understand why those who have been traumatized through the violation of their bodies would come to hate and fear their bodies, or why they would seek to control them by all means possible, even by trying to make them disappear. It's also easy to understand why anorexics with an abusive background would have trouble with sex and intimacy throughout their adult lives.

Irena, age forty-three, had been married for eighteen years and had a fifteen-year-old daughter when she came to see me. Though her reason for seeking treatment was "sexual confusion," a more serious problem was her anorexia and bulimia.

Irena declared up front that she wasn't interested in dealing with her eating disorder, which began when she was seventeen, and which was now so much a part of her identity that she wouldn't know who she was without it. Her habit was to chew her food for the flavour, then to spit it out to avoid ingesting any calories. When forced to eat in a restaurant, or when starvation drove her to binge, she would purge into the nearest toilet bowl afterward. She had been doing this about four times a day for twenty-five years. She would also spend hours burning calories on cardio machines, afraid to allow her five-foot-four body to weigh more than ninety-five pounds.

The sexual confusion, which Irena *was* willing to acknowledge, seriously affected her relationship with her husband, Darren. Though she was ferociously jealous if he looked at another woman, she made him beg for sex. Then, after she had given in to his pleading, she felt like a hooker. Irena also admitted that her bingeing and purging was a functional way of avoiding sex with Darren.

Irena developed a close friendship with her neighbour, Eleanor, a needy and vulnerable divorcee with a two-year-old son. Out of curiosity and boredom, the two began a sexual relationship. Now Irena, who had felt dead inside, experienced an awakening. Her eating disorder subsided for a while as she transferred her addiction from food to an addiction for sex with Eleanor.

After Darren found out about this affair, he said he was also attracted to Eleanor, and the sexual relationship became a threesome. Irena often felt possessive of Eleanor and jealous over Darren; however, she was able to keep these feelings under control until she discovered that Darren and Eleanor were meeting on the sly for trysts, even while both pretended that their main attraction was to Irena.

Now that the threesome was out of Irena's control, her eating disorder took over with renewed vengeance. This was the point when Irena came to see me — not because of her anorexia but because Eleanor had broken off her relationships with both Irena and Darren.

Irena was a Russian-born orphan adopted at age three by a pair of young Canadian professionals. Though she had been affected emotionally by unhappy events before her adoption, she was not able to put these memories into words. As busy professionals, Irena's adoptive parents left her in the hands of a succession of nannies as well as an aunt with whom Irena formed a close bond. This aunt, later diagnosed as bipolar, sexually abused Irena and threatened her with the loss of her love and affection if Irena ever told anyone about the abuse.

Imago Relationship Therapy recognizes that we are likely to be attracted to partners who remind us of both the positives and the negatives of our childhood. The giving and receiving of love (or the not receiving of it) is something that we first learn from our caretakers. Our way of responding to them shapes our expectations as well as the choices we later make and the actions we take to fulfill those expectations.

Imago is the Latin word for "image." Though we may have a fairly detailed conscious image of who we are looking for in a mate, we also have an unconscious list of characteristics, based on what is familiar, that may contradict our conscious values. Even relationships that are abusive or that appear unsuitable to others may feel strangely safe. Sometimes we become stuck in them, and sometimes we use their familiar conflicts for healing and growth. The more extreme the childhood trauma, the more usual for its victims to invite into their adult lives people who will cause them to relive it, either to reinforce their sense of victimhood or as an opportunity to work through their pain and confusion to arrive at their own authenticity.

Through therapy, Irena was able to connect Eleanor's gentle yet hungry sexual touch with the often tender touch of her aunt. Layered over these positive feelings were guilt and shame and betrayal of trust, which Eleanor also revived. These were the painful feelings Irena used to build strong sexual barriers against Darren; at the same time, she was unable to resist Eleanor's sexual allure and neediness, just as she had been powerless to reject her aunt.

Imago Relationship Therapy is most often used for couples. Currently, Darren and Irena are living apart while they decide whether or not their marriage can, or should, be saved. Aside from the issues of trust between them, Irena is trying to determine whether her sexual future lies with men or women or both.

My main concern with Irena is her eating disorder and her body's need for nourishment. At my suggestion, she has also replaced her severe cardio workouts with healing massages.

When dealing with the complexity of anorexia, it's encouraging to remember that while the danger is very real, the majority of anorexics who seek treatment do recover.

CHAPTER 11

OBESITY:
THE FAT OF THE LAND

In recent years, obesity in Western culture has increasingly been represented as an epidemic.

According to "Weighing the Effects and Risks of Obesity" (*Toronto Star*, November 14, 2013), more than 24 percent of Canadian adults identify as obese. U.S. statistics peg that number at 34 percent for adults aged twenty to seventy-four. Given the increase in the number of overweight children, these figures are expected to rise, along with such diseases as type 2 diabetes.

Physical causes of obesity typically cited are cheap, fat-rich foods, sugary drinks, frequent snacking, erratic meal patterns, fewer family meals, and a decrease in exercise. Added to these are the psychological causes: cultural pressures, along with family dysfunction, which encourage restricting and bingeing. In a 2005 study involving 13,640 adults conducted by the University of Toronto schools of social work and public health, entitled "Carrying the Pain of Abuse," women from physically abusive families were found to have a 35 percent greater risk of obesity.

Even much subtler forms of family abuse can have a serious impact on the vulnerable adolescent psyche. In "Shared Risk and Protective Factors for Overweight and Disordered Eating in Adolescents" (*American Journal of Preventative Medicine*, 2007), girls who were teased by family members were found to be one and a half times more likely to engage in binge eating and extreme weight-control behaviours five years later.

Overweight and obese children are also more likely to be bullied by their peers. In a survey of adolescents in grades seven to twelve, 30 percent of girls and 25 percent of boys reported being teased by peers ("Associations of Weight-Based Teasing and Emotional Wellbeing Among Adolescents," *Archives of Pediatrics and Adolescent Medicine*, 2003). Even more of the surveyed girls reported being teased at home.

The so-called "entertainment" media excels in ridiculing anyone it deems too fat, creating and exaggerating eating disorders in those they target. As the world watched, Diana, Princess of Wales, transformed from a young woman of normal weight into a slender fashion icon suffering from bulimia. Her chunky sister-in-law, Sarah Ferguson, the Duchess of York, found herself dubbed the Duchess of Pork. At a time when Kate Middleton, the Duchess of Cambridge, was being described by the media as too thin, the Italian fashion magazine *Grazia* whittled down her waist still further in a cover shot. For this, the editors were soundly rebuked by Buckingham Palace.

It's not just princesses and movie stars who are singled out by the Fat Police. Female Olympians who win gold medals, which requires energy, muscle strength, and stamina, must also pass the tape-measure test.

In the lead-up to the 2012 London Olympic Games, Australian swimmer Leisel Jones, an eight-time medallist, was treated to a tsunami of nasty publicity when a Melbourne newspaper, the *Herald Sun*, ran a photo of her with the caption "Is Leisel Jones too fat or merely fit?" and then asked readers to vote.

Britain's Hollie Avil, the 2007 European and world junior triathlon champion, was forced to retire from competition because of a full-blown eating disorder brought on by a coach's remark about her weight. "Before that, I never even knew what a calorie was," Avil commented. Her weight loss interfered with her buoyancy in the water and weakened her so severely during running and cycling events that she was forced to drop out of the 2008 Summer Olympics.

According to a Norwegian study, 20 percent of elite female athletes meet the criteria for having an eating disorder, compared to 9 percent of females in the general population used as controls ("Prevalence of Eating Disorders in Elite Athletes Is Higher Than in the General Population," *Clinical Journal of*

Sport Medicine, 2004). Not surprisingly, females competing in aesthetic sports like dance, gymnastics, and figure skating were found to be at highest risk.

For those interested in weight loss, the "experts" offer a ridiculous range of possibilities. There's the grapefruit diet, the pineapple diet, the high-fat diet, the Mediterranean diet, the Scarsdale diet, the cabbage soup diet, the South Beach diet, the no-carb diet, the Paleo diet, the green-tea diet, the Wheat Belly diet, the Atkins diet, the liquid diet, and the fasting diet. There are "miracle" diet pills, supplements, and injections — some to boost energy, some to burn fat, some to suppress the appetite. Add to these the diet programs offered by Weight Watchers, Jenny Craig, and Canada's own Dr. Bernstein.

In 2007, Marketdata, Inc. estimated the U.S. diet industry to be worth $58 billion and predicted 6 percent annual growth to $68.7 billion by 2010. The analysis included ten major segments of the U.S. diet industry: diet drugs, diet books and exercise videos, diet soft drinks, artificial sweeteners, diet dinner entrees and meal replacements, health clubs, diet websites, commercial weight-loss chains and hospital-based programs, kids' weight-loss camps, and bariatric (stomach-reduction) surgeries. Diet soft drinks were listed as having the largest share at 29.5 percent, for a total of $19 billion; bariatric surgeries, which were performed a record 177,000 times in 2006, were listed at $4.4 billion; prescription diet drugs at $459 million.

Canadians also pay billions of dollars for weight-loss products and services, with dieters beginning at an ever earlier age. Perhaps the most remarkable fact about this largely unregulated industry is that its financial success is based on its own failure: the failed hopes of people who keep losing and regaining the same twenty pounds, perhaps even gaining an extra five when they come off their diets.

Numerous research projects support the thesis that dieting leads to both weight gain and eating disorders.

In a three-year study published in 1999 in the *British Medical Journal*, girls fourteen to fifteen years who engaged in strict dieting practices were found to be eighteen times more likely than non-dieters to develop an eating disorder within six months. Girls who dieted moderately were five times more likely to develop an eating disorder within six months.

A 1999 study published in the *Journal of Consulting and Clinical Psychology* reported that adolescent girls who diet are at a 324 percent greater risk for obesity than those who don't.

As a poster girl for weight-loss futility, Oprah Winfrey, the world's most famous yo-yo dieter, for decades attracted as much press for her fluctuating weight as for her championing of social issues. Eventually, even she refused to believe in one more magical weight-loss scheme, instead embracing her stylishly dressed ample figure.

The science behind "diet, gain weight" is explained by the body's evolutionary need to store fat as a survival tactic, hard-wired at a time in human development when eating depended on hunting down a woolly mammoth. Starvation causes the body to conserve energy and to hold on to fatty tissue. Likewise, when we gain weight, our bodies adapt to our new size and want to remain there. It's easy to see the trend here: whether we lose weight or gain it, our bodies don't want to let go of their fat reserves.

Not everyone who restricts their diet becomes a chronic dieter, but when genetics, social pressure, and emotional problems kick in, so can an eating disorder. And while it's hard for dieters to win (meaning, to lose weight), the weight-loss industry always wins. As the ideal figure gets ever skinnier, expect industry profits to grow fatter. Who could have predicted there would be a strong market for size zero?

Sarah brought her seventeen-year-old daughter, Amy, to see me, concerned that Amy had an eating disorder, and seeking family counselling. To prove her point, Sarah insisted that Amy roll up her sleeves. Along with random, self-inflicted slashes, Amy had carved DO NOT EAT into her flesh. Her legs were similarly cut and scarred.

Amy's response was, "Like, yeah, okay, so I cut myself. So what?" She also kept up a tirade of verbal abuse against her mother that included swearing and yelling.

When I spoke to Amy alone, she told me that she hated her parents for divorcing six years ago and for their endless bad-mouthing of each other. Amy and her two siblings were always being forced to choose sides, especially Amy, as the oldest. She yearned to return to the time before her father had left her mother for another woman, when her mother was happy and loved her. Amy repeatedly told me that she now wished her mother were dead.

As we talked, Amy admitted that "the good old days" were not as wonderful as she now wanted to believe. Her father had hit her, choked her, called her a fat pig, and told her she would never amount to anything. Her mother was also quick to slap Amy and her siblings into obedience. Since the divorce, Sarah often indulged in tirades against her children's father, then struck them if they refused to take her side or didn't seem to be listening.

Sarah blamed her own weight gain, triggered by three pregnancies, on her husband's cheating and abandonment. Though Amy was sure that her mother binged and purged, Sarah denied this both to Amy and to me.

A child of eleven at the time of her parents' divorce, Amy had internalized her anger at them. This led to her cutting and restricting and bingeing. Now overweight by about forty pounds on a five-foot-three frame, she insisted that the only thing that mattered to her was becoming thin. She told me that she cut herself to hurt her mother, but that she really wanted to kill herself. My experience told me that she was also trying to siphon off her emotional pain by turning it into physical pain over which she had control.

Amy reported that most of her friends were skinnier than she was, thanks to extreme dieting, purging, and exercise, all of which Amy thought were really cool. She remembered boys being attracted to her before she lost control of her weight, and believed that everything in her life would be better if she got thin, though she couldn't remember being happy when she was thin.

Amy admitted to smoking marijuana daily because it was fun and her friends did it. This increased her appetite, which led to more bingeing and forced vomiting. She wanted her GP to give her a prescription for marijuana to ease what she described as chronic neck pain. Though she insisted she wasn't addicted, it was clear to me that she was a habitual user. She would often arrive for her appointments with me half asleep, as if she were stoned. When Amy's friends told her that cocaine was an appetite suppressant, Amy started snorting it to counteract the appetite stimulation of the marijuana. She refused to see that she had a drug addiction, or to acknowledge its connection to her bingeing and purging.

I was convinced that Amy's neck pain stemmed from her excessive vomiting; therefore, if she dealt with bulimia as her core issue, she wouldn't need the marijuana for pain relief. Amy's situation was critically different from that of patients who seek marijuana to deal with chronic pain associated with diseases like cancer and epilepsy. For them, marijuana of various medical grades is prescribed in order to relax neurotransmitters and alleviate pain on the autoimmune level, providing a valuable lifeline. However, when marijuana is misused to deal with the pain of a mental disorder, it masks the problem and blocks treatment, leading to greater anxiety. This was Amy's circumstance. But she preferred to consider her neck pain as a medical problem for which she deserved the relief that marijuana, and then cocaine, offered.

Amy also had problems with her boyfriend that lowered her self-esteem. She was performing oral sex on demand, though she didn't like it, because she was afraid of losing him if she refused.

It proved fortunate for Amy that I was also treating her mother in family counselling. My initial requirement was that Sarah make a written commitment to me that she would never again physically attack Amy. I also explained that if Amy had been under sixteen, I would have been obliged to call the Children's Aid Society to report Sarah for child abuse.

Since Sarah genuinely did not want to hurt her daughter, she readily agreed to my conditions: that she leave the room whenever her fierce temper caused her to wish to strike Amy; that she breathe slowly and deeply until her body calmed down from its "fight" reflex; and that she question herself as to why she wanted to hurt her daughter instead of nurture her. Since Sarah was a practising Catholic, I also suggested that she work through the Overeaters Anonymous twelve steps, adapting them to her own faith.

Though it was hard for Sarah to take the lead in helping Amy, she stuck to her treatment promises because she loved her daughter. She also acknowledged her own not-so-secret eating disorder, which Amy had been mimicking.

Sarah's change in attitude and behaviour brought about a wonderful flowering in Amy and caused her to shift to the point where she wanted to get better to please both her mother and herself. She also came to realize that her ways of problem solving — restricting, bingeing, smoking marijuana — had increased her unhappiness. At core, Amy and her mother were hungry to embrace and care for each other. The depth of their anger was also a measure of their love.

Since I believe that people suffering from eating disorders should reach out for as many lifelines as possible, I suggested that Amy enter a drug rehabilitation program. I was also pleased when both mother and daughter agreed to follow the food action plan that I outline in the next chapter.

As the story of Amy and Sarah illustrates, when one member of a family has an addiction, another is likely to have a similar trait. This is especially true of mothers and daughters. Fear of food, dieting, bingeing, purging, and over-concern with body image are all learned behaviours.

Even when the disorder is not passed on, every member of a family will be affected. While our society understands the seriousness of drug and alcohol addiction, most people see issues with food as self-invented, requiring only willpower to cure. Concerned parents and partners often have extreme difficulty understanding why the person they love struggles with something as seemingly unthreatening, pleasurable, and basic as food.

An anxious parent who feels responsible for the health of a child may attempt to seize control of the child's eating habits in a way that creates or encourages a disorder. Constantly forcing a child to eat, or emphasizing restriction and body image can cause the child to become more manipulative and deceptive about his or her eating habits.

When dealing with a loved one's eating disorder, never comment on his or her appearance or pass judgment on her behaviour. Avoid accusatory "you" statements that convey shame, blame, guilt, anger, or impatience. Instead of "You're getting too fat for your clothes" or "You need to eat more," say "It scares me to hear you vomiting" or "I'm concerned about you because you eat so little."

Avoid making food the focus of your relationship through nagging. Instead, focus on feelings — the importance of the relationship between you and that person.

At the same time, don't deny the seriousness of bingeing and purging. As soon as you become aware of a disorder, persuade your loved one to go to a medical doctor to establish an appropriate weight for his or her body. Also suggest a rehab or therapeutic program. With eating disorders, no one size fits all. Multiple approaches multiply the chances of success.

CHAPTER 12

YOUR ACTION PLAN:
FROM BINGEING TO RECOVERY

B y now, I hope everyone reading this book understands: *Diets don't work.* This chapter isn't about losing weight so you can become skinny. It's the practical part of a larger plan to help you become a physically healthy, fully realized person.

Like any reputable action plan involving the body, this process begins by urging you to get a medical checkup to discover special needs and individual challenges. Are you taking any medications, such as birth control pills, that perhaps cause weight gain as a side effect? Do you have an underactive thyroid or slow metabolism? What is your blood-sugar level? Do you need vitamin supplements? What is your BMI (body mass index), based on your weight and height? Continuous medical monitoring is desirable for everyone, but it's essential for those who have health problems related to obesity.

A cautionary note: While this chapter contains useful nutritional advice for compulsive overeaters, general guidelines for any eating disorder or addiction are not enough in themselves. Outside support is required. This is especially critical for anorexics. You must be monitored by a medical professional who provides regular checkups to make sure your weight is not decreasing. You will also need intensive therapy to get to the emotional root of why you are endangering your life. I hope that you care enough about yourself and those who love you to make these two intentions the centrepiece of *your* action plan.

Since anyone who has read this far knows my story, you'll understand why I also urge all of you who suspect you may have ADHD, or a mood disorder, to undergo testing. Then, before you decide on a pharmaceutical solution, I suggest that you consult your medical doctor or a naturopath about useful natural remedies like magnesium, omega-3, zinc, and iron, which can be found in health food stores and many drug stores.

Remember, too, that with neurological conditions like ADHD, an important part of subverting self-sabotage is self-awareness. Strive to be your own best friend when it comes to recognizing the onset of impulsive and hyperactive behaviours. Sometimes when I'm talking, so many different thoughts start shooting off in different directions that it's hard for me to stay on topic. If I feel comfortable in my surroundings, I may say aloud to those around me, "Sorry, my ADHD is taking over." More often, I just slow myself down, then calmly sort my thoughts in terms of relevance and importance. I also remind myself that my ADHD is a welcome part of what makes me unique.

Whenever you find your thoughts spinning, I recommend this combination of self-awareness and a mindful pause. Often this is enough to create a mental shift in your neurological pathways that will allow your more rational self to regain control.

YOUR ACTION PLAN

This plan to counter binge eating isn't just about food. It's also about your feelings, thoughts, and behaviours surrounding food. It's simple, straightforward, and designed for success, if you remain committed. The best way you can make it work for yourself is to give up any desperate, fear-based desire to control your body, or to judge it by how many pounds you lose in a day or a week. As humans, we cannot control the precise outcome of any situation, or even any moment, whether it has to do with the food we eat or a relationship we're in. We can, however, control our actions and our thought patterns to bring about our highest good. Forget about the numbers on your weight scale — in fact, forget about weighing yourself at all.

Only by letting go of these futile mind-based attempts at control can you gain genuine control through listening to your body and paying attention to its real needs.

Yes, your shadow in the form of your addiction will sometimes hamper your efforts. It will lie to you to persuade you to give in to your cravings. But remember that it's only your enemy for as long as you allow it to be. It was, after all, your shadow that brought you on this journey. It's your shadow that you may want to thank when you discover how much stronger and more confident you are becoming. When I'm talking to clients, I'm often aware of my shadow sitting on my shoulder, reminding me of how much I've learned because of it, and how much I now have to share.

Think of your action plan as a lifestyle change rather than as a way of coping with your disorder, then allow yourself to become excited about where it will lead you. Remember the severity of my disorder and my years of uncontrolled bingeing and purging. If I could crawl out from under my ice-cream mountain, you can, too!

So, let's begin …

Make a binge list

Include any and all of the dangerous foods — one bite, and you want ten more — that "trigger" you. Typically, these are processed foods rich in fats and sugar, but some are more deceptive. Perhaps they possess a salt content that has you reaching for a sugary drink (think potato chips). Your list is individual to you. It may even contain foods generally considered healthy. For some people, salad can become a trigger once they load it up with high-fat, sugary dressing. Same with broccoli and kale, well salted and slathered with butter. Nothing is exempt from what we bingers will choose as a food to numb our feelings. One of my clients ate so many carrots that her skin turned orange from the carotene. Another binged on powdered milk. That's why this list is individual to *you*. As you gain more insight into your addiction, expect to add other culprits.

Eat three meals a day

This is the core of your recovery. Each meal should fill an entire twelve-inch plate but should not overflow it. Anything you eat beyond this is stolen food — you sabotaging you. Here's the good news: You can eat anything you want as long as it is not on your binge list. Remember what happened to me when I ate pasta every day for four months? Nothing, as far as my weight was concerned, but very important changes took place in my head and in my emotions. I was losing my love–hate relationship to food and creating a platform of stability that would allow me to stop victimizing myself. One reminder: If, for example, you're allowed bread, that does NOT mean you can place a loaf on a twelve-inch plate, then stack it with butter and call it a meal just because it doesn't overflow. My clients often giggle when I tell them this, but having been a binger myself, I know this is the sort of self-defeating trick obsessive overeaters play on themselves in order to hold tightly to their addiction.

Never leave your house without knowing where and when you will have your three meals. If that means bagging a lunch, then do so. Treat this rule as if your life depended on it, which it very well might.

Pay attention to the kinds of situations that make you want to over-indulge or restrict, and try to eliminate them from your routine — a route home that takes you past an ice-cream parlour, a break from work in which you feel you need to reward yourself, an all-you-can-eat buffet that makes you think you're not getting your money's worth unless you return for seconds or include a trip to the dessert counter.

Be conscious of the fact that you are eating — don't watch TV or read a book or otherwise distract yourself from your meal.

Be sensuously aware of *what* you're eating. Admire the food on your plate — the colours, the shapes. Chew your food thoroughly and slowly. Enjoy its smell, its taste, its texture. Be aware of its function — to nurture your body and provide you with energy. Too many people who claim to love food obsess about it except when they are actually eating. Then, they bolt and stuff it down so they can start fantasizing about their next fix.

Eat one or two snacks a day

These snacks are planned, not random, and it's your choice as to whether you have one or two per day. Your snack can be a granola bar or yogurt, an apple or a banana — a single portion of anything you enjoy that isn't on your binge list. Choose a time when you usually feel low-energy, or when you're likely to experience the most temptation, such as when co-workers break to enjoy a snack. When I first began this recovery program, I chose to have only one snack a day. Some days I ate two because I felt I needed a second uplift, but this was always planned, not a decision made impulsively.

Be aware of what you're feeling while you're eating

This is a huge part of your recovery that we'll talk more about later.

When you've finished your food, take a minute to experience the pleasant sensation of being full and to feel grateful for it.

Never restrict

If you lapse, don't punish yourself by restricting at your next meal or the next day. Instead, forgive yourself and continue with your three meals and snacks.

Don't panic or use one lapse as an excuse to go on a week-long binge. Remember, your shadow is a tempter who speaks to you from your addict's brain. You may have lost this one battle, but you haven't lost the war. See this moment as an opportunity to be stronger the next time around.

Keep in mind that this is a trial-and-error process — an attempt to find what works for *you*. Perfection is not part of the process, nor is it the goal.

Keep a food diary

This is an optional step but also a very useful one. It helps you to determine which foods leave you satiated and satisfied, and which foods leave you hungry and vulnerable to a binge. List everything that you eat — no cheating — along with the portion size, but don't keep track of calories.

Try for a balanced diet

We all know that fruits, vegetables, protein, and whole grains are healthy for us, whereas sugary, fried, processed, and white-flour foods are not. Once you have stabilized your three-meal, two-snack program, consider substituting more of the healthier foods — not in the spirit of martyrdom but because you're willing to expand your taste palate.

Conquer your fear of food

Give up the notion that if you eat what you want you'll automatically become fat. It's the starving and bingeing that mess up your metabolism and cause your body to protectively store fat because it fears you will keep starving it. Sometimes we avoid foods we enjoy, such as potatoes, because we believe they'll make us fat when, in fact, they could be part of a balanced diet. Challenge yourself by eating foods that you have stigmatized as long as they are not on your "danger" list. Once my diet became more moderate and my body knew it was no longer going to be starved, it let go of the weight I thought I could never lose without restricting. Also be aware that, over time, your list will change. Eventually — perhaps after many years — you will overcome all your fear of food. More about that later.

Eating awareness

What your body wants and what your addicted mind wants are two very different things. In order to override your addiction, it's necessary to get in touch with your emotions, thoughts, and desires both before and after bingeing, either to prevent a relapse or to at least put more time between this binge and the next.

Dealing with temptation

How typical is this situation for you? You catch yourself thinking about one of your danger foods. These thoughts get stronger. You picture it, or maybe it's actually sitting on a table in front of you. Before yielding to temptation, make sure to ask yourself, Why do I want to eat that? What emotion am I feeling? What void am I trying to fill? When circumstances allow, record your answers on paper or on your phone.

This is where I would like to introduce you to a fantastic acronym (a word made up of the first letters of the words it stands for): HALT — Hungry, Angry, Lonely, Tired. As I learned at Overeaters Anonymous, these feelings represent special danger zones for anyone with an addiction.

> **Hungry:** What are you hungry for — a reward? Recognition? Drama? Love? Sex? Freedom from financial worry? Passion? Purpose? How will eating that doughnut solve this problem?

> **Angry:** Did someone annoy you, or are you always on a short fuse? Who are you angry at? Be specific. How will eating those potato chips punish the person who angered you?

> **Lonely:** Is this a temporary feeling, or do you always feel apart from others? Are you planning to make that piece of cake your new best friend? I doubt that it will repay the favour.

> **Tired:** Did you have a tough day? Are you depressed or merely bored? How much excitement will that grilled cheese sandwich add to your life?

If none of these big four reflect your mood, check through your typical emotions: *Am I jealous — of whom and why? Do I hate myself — just now, or all the time? Am I feeling powerless?* Keep going until you find the right emotional fit, then ask yourself how the food that you are currently craving will solve that problem.

Go back further in time, most likely to childhood, then ask yourself, When did I learn to regard food as a reward and its restriction as a punishment? Who taught me that? Who and what reinforced that view? Since your "reward" foods are most likely the ones that now cause you to binge, ask yourself, Did being given those foods as a reward actually do me a favour? Did I mistakenly come to regard those foods as a sub-stitute for love?

Food is energy. Food is nurture. Feel grateful for food as a blessing, but ask yourself, How can food that is damaging my body be love? Connecting food to love and reward makes a false association. The same is true in regard to food as "comfort." Comfort is what we get from people we like and love, from a walk in the woods on a beautiful day, from a warm fire in winter, or from our accomplishments, not from a piece of fudge cake!

If after all this, you can't shift away from the desires of your addicted brain, ask yourself, If I do binge, how will I feel afterward? You know the answer to that: guilty, remorseful, ashamed, panicky, weak, defeated, like a failure, lacking in self-esteem, et cetera. So, is it worth it? Does that piece of fudge cake, followed by a binge on pecan pie, really feel like "love," "com-fort," or a "reward" for being a good girl or boy?

Once you put yourself in touch with your feelings, you can often shift your consciousness far enough to stop a binge in its tracks. If you do relapse, then enjoy your treat as a conscious choice, not as the guilty act of an addict on automatic pilot.

While this process of self-questioning may at first seem lengthy, even-tually you will sniff out the emotions that typically fuel your binges so that your absence from a party or the dinner table while you escape to the wash-room to deal with your dilemma won't happen as often or be as noticeable.

So, you caved in and you binged — now what? First, give yourself the ben-efit of the doubt. Ask yourself:

- Did I binge because I was genuinely hungry?
- Did I eat enough at my last meal?
- Did I have enough carbohydrates and fibre to feel full?
- Do I need to make adjustments to my meal plan?
- Should I plan two snacks instead of one?

If you have no reasonable or practical excuse for your binge, don't beat yourself up. Forgive yourself, then go back to your three-meals-and-two-snacks food plan. Guilt and shame are not useful emotions except as a prod to modify your behaviour in order to avoid them.

ESTABLISH LIFELINES

As the Beatles put it, *I get by with a little help from my friends.* When suffering from a food addiction, it's important to be able to reach out to someone whom you can trust during times of high temptation. Perhaps this will be a family member or a close friend who understands what you are going through, or someone in a buddy group formed with others to support each other. Perhaps it will be your therapist, who has agreed to be on call, or a sponsor from Overeaters Anonymous. The best mentor is someone who has recovered from an eating disorder, and remember, OA offers free counselling and has chapters worldwide. Since your lifeline is someone who has agreed to support you, phone, text, or email that person when your addict's mind threatens to take over. And given the fact that no one can be available 24–7, it's important to have more than one human you can count on.

Let me be even more explicit: I doubt the action plan or food plan could work without support. I have had clients do well for a while going it alone, only to return a few weeks later to insist that the plan "doesn't work." What didn't work was their failure to put in place some kind of support system to keep themselves accountable. That's like investing 50 percent and expecting a 100 percent return. Your addiction will win. You *need* lifelines. They are a critical part of the action plan, not just a suggestion.

Here are the kinds of situations in which I urge you to reach out for support:

- You are at a party and all you can think about is the wonderful buffet filled with your trigger foods. You have only to pick up a plate, like everyone else, and load it.
- You are home alone in front of your TV, exhausted from a bad day, bored, and lonely. Your addict's brain is telling you that all you need to feel better is to go into the kitchen and treat yourself to a small snack.

- Someone angered you, arousing the irrational belief that if you reward yourself by bingeing, you will somehow get back at that person.

A second lifeline to keep you grounded is an emergency journal — a notebook or an electronic device that stays with you wherever you go, into which you can pour your thoughts and feelings. Seeing your emotions written out helps you to be more objective in assessing your addict brain's sly deceptions.

A third lifeline is an affirmation that you repeat to yourself, not only when struggling with your addiction but also when you're feeling strongest or when you're going about your ordinary business not feeling much at all: *Because I love and respect my body, I will nurture and keep it from harm.*

A fourth lifeline is your willingness to take action in difficult situations. This can mean something simple like leaving the scene of your temptation for a few minutes to switch your neurological channel by taking a few deep breaths or perhaps reciting the Serenity Prayer: *Grant me the serenity to accept the things I cannot change, the courage to change the things I can, and the wisdom to know the difference. Thy will, not mine, be done.* If you have a religious affiliation, you may wish to pray for help to your god or higher power.

A fifth lifeline is avoidance. You know from experience — especially thanks to your journal — that certain situations and certain people cause you to binge. These may be people you love, and who love you, but perhaps on some unconscious level they're sabotaging you, or causing you to sabotage yourself. Take a temporary leave of absence from these situations and relationships until you get a grip on whatever it is that's undermining you. Treat this as an emergency until that wonderful time when it ceases to be an emergency. Refrain from blame either way. Just do it.

A sixth lifeline is matching your meal preparation to what is best for curbing your addiction. Often, binge eaters are completely disconnected from the process of shopping and preparing meals. For them, learning to read labels, be creative with recipes, and experiment with spices can aid their recovery. For addicts who already spend too much time shopping and preparing food, the opposite solution is best: Try to stay out of grocery stores and the kitchen as much as possible by delegating or trading off those tasks to others.

A seventh lifeline is exercise. No need to overdo it. Whether you choose yoga, Pilates, weightlifting, walking, or climbing stairs — do just enough so that you can feel your muscles stretch and lengthen within whatever fat you may be carrying. Since I enjoy exercising, I usually work out three or five days a week for forty-five minutes, unless I'm travelling or not feeling up to par, in which case I might not work out at all. As with food, I listen to what my body wants. I used to feel guilty about doing less than five days of sixty minutes, but not any more. I mainly lift weights. I also sprint six times for thirty-second intervals, one or two times a week. Only rarely do I do thirty minutes of cardio because, frankly, I hate to sweat (partly because it messes up my long hair — my girlie side again!).

An eighth lifeline is sleep. You need enough for your system. For most people, this is about seven and a half hours. If you're tired, your judgment about food is impaired, you exercise less, your metabolism is slower, and your hormones are affected. This means that your body will produce more of the hormone ghrelin, which tells you to eat, and less of the hormone leptin, which tells you to stop eating. The result? Weight gain, of course.

A ninth lifeline is maintaining a self-supportive attitude. Forgive yourself for the hold that your addiction has had on you, and may still have on you. Forgive others whom you blame for causing your problem, or enabling it, or failing to understand it. Believe in yourself, accept yourself, do your best, and be optimistic about the outcome.

GETTING BETTER

During my recovery, I experienced a conflict between the Overeaters Anonymous idea that trigger foods are forever off limits, and the clinical view that all foods, in proper proportion, should become part of a normal diet. After following the OA guidelines for a number of years, I personally found I could make friends with, or simply ignore, my trigger foods. It took me a very long time to arrive at this position, and the approach doesn't work for everyone.

Once you reach the point in your recovery when you can distinguish real hunger from emotional hunger, you may be ready and able to start introducing your trigger foods in small quantities.

Peanut butter was once at the top of my danger list, because I knew that if I ate a spoonful, I would eat the entire jar, then possibly binge for a couple of weeks. This, of course, made peanut butter super scary. One day, when I felt secure in my understanding of myself and my addict's brain, I decided to reintroduce peanut butter (the peanut-only kind, with no additives). After spreading it on my breakfast toast, I was tempted to have more but controlled that urge because I knew I could have more the next day if I wanted.

That idea of "deferred pleasure" enabled me to put the jar in the cupboard for the first time in my life. I still harboured thoughts of taking it out, but every day that I stopped at one serving, my "no" muscle grew stronger. The reason? I was no longer depriving myself or allowing my addict's brain to convince me that if I didn't eat the whole jar now, I might never have peanut butter again. Today, when I spread it on my toast, I can sit next to the jar for the rest of the meal without even thinking of dipping in a spoon.

Sometimes when you reintroduce binge foods, the unexpected happens. After three friends and I had enjoyed a very satisfying meal at a good restaurant, one woman insisted on ordering a chocolate dessert to be shared among the four of us. It was exactly the sort of cake I used to binge on — rich and dense. Though I didn't want it, the other women kept bugging me to share their guilt. Normally, that wouldn't have persuaded me, but I was at a stage where I felt confident enough to take a chance. Since the dessert wasn't large, I ended up with about two bites on my plate. The chocolate tasted as delicious as I remembered, but after I'd swallowed a forkful, I could feel that it didn't agree with my digestive system, so I pushed aside the other piece and forgot about it. These decadent desserts now remain on my "no" list — not because I'm afraid of them, but because my body no longer wants them. I probably couldn't even digest a full serving, which — after the enormous quantities I once ate — still amazes me. Perhaps I built up an intolerance because of overindulgence. Perhaps my body has such painful memories of purging that it refuses to digest this type of food.

Be optimistically aware that what has happened to me will also happen to you if you stick to your action plan. Over time, your list of taboo foods will change. Eventually, you may overcome all your fear of food as I have done, so that you can eat in moderation everything that was once on your list. You may still have sensitivities to food that your body no longer wants, but you will no longer have fear. This happens because once you get to the root of why you have been abusing food, you will no longer need it as a numbing substance. You will enjoy food for the sensuous pleasure that it brings. Life itself will satiate your deep emotions.

MY ACTION PLAN

People often ask what I, as a former addict, eat now. Though I'm happy to answer that question, I emphasize that what works for me won't necessarily work for others in the same way, though some of my choices may provide a useful guide. The quantities I list are approximate, since I never weigh, measure, or attempt to count calories or control portions — those were the training wheels I required for many years because of my food addiction. As you will see, I eat a lot.

Breakfast

- 2 organic eggs cooked in either coconut oil or butter
- 2 slices of gluten-free toast made either from brown rice or buckwheat, spread with coconut oil or butter
- 1 piece of fruit, either a banana or grapefruit
- 1 glass of freshly squeezed green juice, composed of mostly seasonal organic vegetables — kale, radishes, carrots, spinach, celery, dandelion greens, cucumber, beets, beet greens, parsley, ginger, garlic, and a lemon

or

- 2 slices of Ezekiel cinnamon raisin toast and an organic nut butter spread without additives, plus a cup of banana with cinnamon

Lunch

- brown-rice pasta with meat sauce — a generous bowl, about two cups cooked

or

- 1 full chicken breast
- ½ cup of cooked kasha with coconut oil
- a generous bowl of salad with olive oil, salt, pepper, and spices

Snack

- a handful of raw nuts, a piece of fruit, or a treat such as a dessert made from soaked nuts, honey, coconut, avocado, cocoa

Dinner

- steak or chicken or hamburger, always organic if home-cooked (or a source of vegetarian protein such as tofu or tempeh)
- ½ cup to ¾ cup quinoa or brown rice, or squash or sweet potato
- a green vegetable such as broccoli, or a freshly squeezed green juice

or

- chicken breast dipped in egg, breaded with rice bread crumbs, and fried in coconut oil, served with broccoli and lentils

Snack

- sometimes after dinner, nuts or fruit, occasionally a treat; see previous snack list

A cautionary note: When I incorporate sweets, such as chocolate and coconut ice cream, I sometimes begin to crave more as in the old days, even though my stomach doesn't feel well, and my skin might break out the next day. I believe this type of craving is also hormone related, since it corresponds with my menstrual periods.

It takes time and patience to find out what your body needs and wants, after years of abuse, and often this changes with time. I now know that I'm overly sensitive to milk, sugar, and gluten, and paradoxically, the more I consume them, the more I crave them. When I stay away from them, the cravings end and I feel better mentally, emotionally, and physically. Today I eat sweets, but only ones that are natural and reasonably healthy — manuka honey, dark chocolate, natural nut butters, raw desserts made from nutritious foods such as avocados, dates, cocoa, coconut, figs, strawberries, blueberries, kale chips, carob chips, and sweet potatoes.

Since my meal plan provides me with lots of energy, I also stay clear of all so-called energy drinks, including coffee. As a daily supplement, I do take one tablespoon of fish oil to get omega-3.

As I've said, your lifetime meal plan is a matter of trial and error, just as mine is. There is no "right" solution, and lifestyle changes, such as travel, may require you to make creative substitutions.

THE BALANCING ACT

If you eat a healthy, balanced diet, your body will find its own set-point weight. This will depend on your height, bone structure, muscle mass, and so on. I was surprised to find that my set point was what I used to regard as my skinniest weight — probably around 120 pounds on my five-foot-five frame. I can't be sure because I haven't weighed myself for many years. I'm happy as long as my jeans fit!

My clients are often afraid — as I used to be — that their set-point weight will be higher than they ideally want it to be. Here's the thing: Society admires a wide range of facial features — different complexions, hair colour, eye colour; facial shapes from round to triangular, from oval to oblong; high cheekbones or dimples; wide mouths or rosebuds; noses that are pert or aquiline — depending on how these are assembled.

In contrast, our culture insists that our bodies, which are less flexible than our faces, be of a certain type — an ideal that may change within a single lifetime. The Victorians liked forward-thrusting chests and derrieres exaggerated by bustles. The twenties liked their flat-chested, bob-haired flappers; the forties their wartime pin-up girls with big breasts, small waists, long legs, and long hair. Since the sixties, fashion has favoured the elongated, ever-more-slender figure, as if women could be stretched on one of those medieval torture machines. You can't do this to real women, but you can do this to their photographs, and then persuade real women that this is how they should look.

Whether your body type corresponds to the current fashion depends on factors well beyond your control. Self-acceptance is the greatest gift you can give yourself. Next time you look at a fashion magazine, ask yourself if you really want to go back to restricting and purging, as those models probably must do, just to get rid of ten more pounds, knowing you'll probably put fifteen back on. Always remember, your body is right for you, while the fickle fashion ideal is quite likely wrong. Men don't necessarily prefer the slimmest, tallest women, either. Just as often, they choose a more curvaceous, cuddlier body type possessed by someone who radiates poise and confidence and has more on her mind than her appearance. That choice is within your control, because what really matters is how you feel about yourself.

Change — even for the better — can be challenging. Take it one step at time. Stick to the plan, and you'll eventually get where you want to go. Remember: You are far more than just your eating disorder.

CHAPTER 13

SEX:
FINDING THE ON SWITCH

Nineteen-year-old Maya, of Chinese descent, came to see me because of family problems. Her mother had died of cancer when Maya was only three months old, and she had been brought up by her grandmother, who was now dying of leukemia. Since her two older siblings had married, Maya was left alone to provide palliative care for her grandmother. Maya's father, the family's hard-working breadwinner, was often harsh and angry with Maya.

Maya had a severe eating disorder brought on by stress. Because she couldn't control anything else in her life, she attempted to control her intake of food on a strict cycle. For two days she would binge, then purge by vomiting; for the next five days, she would refuse to eat for as long as she could, then chew and spit out her food to get the taste without the calories; next, she would eat frozen food with little flavour so as not to trigger a binge; then, she would eat out of the garbage because that food was even less appealing. After that, Maya felt she had earned her binge, and she would restart her cycle.

During her first appointment, Maya told me that she had never been kissed by a boy because she was saving herself for marriage. A month later, she began to date twenty-five-year-old Sidney. That's when it became clear that underlying her romantic fantasy of saving her virginity was not only a fear of sex but also a fear of being touched and of being seen naked. Maya hated her body, which she considered fat, though her weight was within normal limits. She didn't mind touching Sidney as long as she was fully clothed, and on days when she was providing him with sexual stimulation, she was able to eat more normally. At least, at first. When Sidney began to pressure her for sex, Maya's bingeing worsened, and her attempts at control became more futile.

After Maya and Sidney had been dating fourteen months, Sidney delivered an ultimatum: either give him sex or he was leaving. This led to a rough encounter that Maya experienced as rape, and that created symptoms of PTSD that had to be addressed therapeutically. Sidney excused his roughness on the grounds that Maya had made him wait too long. He also told her that he'd been seeing other, more compliant women, and that now he wanted to break off his relationship with Maya. Around that same time, Maya's grandmother died. Maya's feelings over her grandmother's death were intensified by Sidney's abandonment, and her eating disorder worsened.

Though Sidney was the wrong mate for Maya in terms of providing happiness, he was the right mate for creating a crisis that forced her to either rescue or destroy herself. His harshness mirrored Maya's father's treatment of her, and his abandonment brought into focus her mother's early abandonment of her through death and now the loss of her grandmother.

Before Maya could listen to her body's nutritional needs, or experience sexual fulfillment, she needed to release her body from the task of storing pain and swallowing stress. This meant allowing herself to grieve — for her unknown mother, for her grandmother, for the loss of a man she had hoped would love her. Grieving is a natural, healthy reaction to loss. In my view, there is no such thing as too many tears. People who don't grieve end up repeating the same experience of loss and abandonment with different people, and perhaps, like Maya, develop an addiction to distract themselves from their pain.

Grieving dissolved Maya's barriers of distrust sufficiently to let the work of healing begin. Because of what I felt were blocks in Maya's body, I decided to ask her permission to try energy work with her. All thoughts and emotions interact with the body, and blocks are created by unconscious choices that usually are forced rather than free. Perhaps these choices were once necessary for survival. Perhaps they were created through our own misconceptions, or the misconceptions of those on whom we once relied.

Energy healing is a technique that I use to bypass the mind in order to access the wisdom of the body. It begins by putting the client into a state of total relaxation. To do this, I dim the lights, then make sure that the client is physically comfortable, either sitting in an easy chair or lying down with cushions and a blanket, whichever feels safest to him or her. Since Maya was lying down, I asked if I could touch her shoulder for a moment to connect my energy with hers, to find my own quiet space, and to ask the universe to guide me in fulfilling my intention of serving her highest good.

I then asked Maya to close her eyes and to take a few deep breaths. In a brief meditation, I suggested that she pack all her daily concerns and worries, one by one, into a bubble that she would then place beside her. While this was happening, I moved my hands around Maya without touching her, feeling her energy and using my intuition to sweep, brush, and otherwise clear away stale or negative energy. Since this process is entirely experiential and relies completely on the trust of the client and the intuition of the therapist, it is difficult to explain, but Maya later reported, as most of my clients do, that it made her feel less burdened and lighter.

Once Maya and I were in sync on the deepest level, I asked her to select one of the problems from her bubble, to focus on it, and then to travel mentally and emotionally into the part of her body that hurt. After a few moments, Maya replied, "There's something in my stomach, and it's black. It looks like a cloud — no, it's heavier than a cloud. It's something dense ..."

In a voice that was at first tentative, then gained in confidence, Maya answered my questions, eventually identifying the black cloud as a fetus in her mother's body. That fetus was Maya, which she located in the stomach because as a child, she thought that's where babies came from.

Since Maya's mother had died so soon after Maya's birth, and since Maya's father was always so angry with her, Maya came to believe, as a child, that she was responsible for her mother's death. Since this thought was lodged deep in her unconsciousness, she had no way of correcting it as an adult.

Because of the intensity of this work, it's always necessary to ground clients when they come out of a session. Sitting up and opening their eyes is a slow process because they feel as if they are returning from a different dimension, to which I travelled with them. Sometimes I suggest they tap their feet to ground themselves. Sometimes I gently push them forward by one shoulder to make sure they are stable, then have them drink a glass of water.

I never know how a session will end, and I'm always amazed at how uniquely transformational each one becomes, not only for the client but also for me. Afterward, I always feel rested, as if I've slept for hours.

Bringing Maya's false information from the past into present awareness was a huge step for her. She still has a romantic view of her future, which includes marriage and having three children. She has a long way to go to heal her adult body through proper nutrition, which means giving up restricting and bingeing. Only then will she be able to fully enjoy the pleasures of intimacy and sex.

My familiarity with clients like Maya, along with my own experience, has taught me the profound physical and emotional connection between food and sex. This is especially true for women, since both eating and sex involve allowing something "foreign" into our bodies. If we abuse the body as an object of dislike and distrust, then these negative emotions are easily projected onto the "invaders."

Both eating and intercourse are biologically designed to provide pleasure as well as fulfill basic drives. If food becomes our source of comfort, we will use it to feed our psychological wounds, so that sex will not be a priority. It might not even be on our radar. Instead, our craving for love, for being touched and caressed, will be transferred to the desire for a piece of apple pie or a fix of ice cream, both of which are easier to access as instant gratification.

Similarly, if food — the most basic of our survival needs — becomes an arena of suffering instead of pleasure, then pleasure itself becomes tainted as something to be avoided rather than sought out and experienced. Fear of food becomes fear of sex. When food addiction is the cover for childhood sexual abuse, then the order can be reversed: Fear of sex becomes fear of food. Unconsciously, the damaged psyche may want to pile on the pounds to create a fortress in which to hide: *Now I'm safe because no one will want me.* The traumatized victim has no understanding of setting boundaries beyond *No — go away! I am not a sex object.* The inability to set boundaries may also be transferred to food, resulting in bingeing and restricting. That is when our bodies may move so far out of our conscious awareness that they become dangerous to us through the conditions of morbid obesity or anorexia and require both medical and psychological intervention to be restored to health. Even a less severe food addiction can create abdominal distress and fluctuations in body weight that can disturb our hormone levels and deaden our libidos.

A distorted body image is another reason for sexual disinterest. Even people of normal weight, such as Maya, often see fat — the culturally inspired enemy — where it doesn't exist. Though the image is false, the shame is very real.

Getting into bed with someone when all you can think about is your fat thighs doesn't feel sexy for you, and your awkward discomfort will soon telegraph itself to your partner. Even when the worst of an eating disorder is over, the habit of self-doubt often continues: *Am I "perfect" enough?*

Food and sex are alike in that they intimately involve all five senses: taste, touch, smell, sight, hearing. When issues with food or sex have made these senses dangerous, they are likely to be turned off in all areas of life. For those of us with a sexual disorder, opening ourselves to the sensual pleasures of sex can begin with opening ourselves to the sensuous pleasures of food.

As we have already discussed in the action plan, when we are most present during mealtime, we use our eyes to admire the colour and shape of the food on our plates, our noses to anticipate its flavour, our mouths to experience its different textures, our tongues to taste it, and our ears to hear it crunch as we chew. In this way, we passionately experience food on a primal level.

Compare this with Maya's eating of food that was frozen or taken from the garbage precisely because it was flavourless or disgusting to look at. That was how damaged and disconnected from pleasure her senses had become.

Like food, good sex presents us with a sensuous banquet. Through the eyes of love and desire, our partner's body visually awakens our appetite for fulfillment. Nature has also designed us so that tastes and smells, whether conscious or subliminal like pheromones, become powerful aphrodisiacs. The sounds we make during sex heighten our mutual arousal, while the feel of our partner's hands on our body keeps us intimately and pleasur-ably in the moment. From birth, we all crave to be touched. Without that sensation, a baby cannot survive emotionally. We never lose that need, even though we may bury it under layers of inhibition.

For those of you who have spent your lives disliking your bodies, it may be necessary to remind you of the importance of good grooming, not primarily to attract a partner, but to begin the love affair with yourself. For this, I suggest a program of pampering: soaking in a scented bath rather than taking a quick shower; rubbing yourself with creams and oils; wearing silky lingerie and sleeping in satin sheets; indulging in manicures and pedicures; breathing deeply and consciously so as to draw long drafts of oxygen down into the sex organs; listening to romantic music; and freeing the body through dance, either slow and sentimental or wild and passionate.

How we dress also plays a significant role in how we feel about ourselves and how we want others to treat us. For those who have neglected their appearance, the first step toward feeling sexy may involve ditching the unisex tents, the baggy pants, the freaky hairdos, and hats chosen to conceal or distract. Women who are confident of their sexuality know that makeup exaggerating the lips and eyes, bright fabrics, form-fitting clothes, low necklines, bare arms, flashy fingernails, short skirts, high heels, and glittery accessories are a celebration of their femininity. They also know that party clothes, which emphasize sex and individuality, are quite different from business clothes, which emphasize team-playing and focusing on the job at hand. The more comfortable you feel with your body, the more likely you are to choose clothes that make you feel attractive and appropriate in all situations.

Full body acceptance also means looking at our naked selves in the mirror and embracing, honouring, and respecting what we see. The British TV show *How to Look Good Naked*, which first aired in 2006, persuaded women who felt self-conscious about their bodies to pose for tasteful nude photos that later were blown up and displayed on public billboards or the sides of buildings. Candidates were *not* urged to lose weight or to undergo a physical makeover. Instead, they were put through a series of confidence-building exercises that included viewing a lineup of silhouetted women of various shapes and sizes, then choosing the figure they believed was closest to their own. Almost invariably they chose a silhouette several sizes too large. One candidate's episode ended with her walking, naked, down a catwalk in front of her friends and family!

Our bodies alone are never who we really are. They are just the container for our essential selves. The number-one destroyer of our sexuality is judgment, especially self-judgment. Often we think we are being criticized by others, when in fact it's our own self-sabotaging voice cruelly calling us to account. Remember that wise saying, "What other people think of me is none of my business. What I think of myself is my business." When we look at our bodies we must see our inner beauty radiating through, confident in the knowledge that if that's what we see, others will see it as well.

Full body acceptance also requires us to know and love our genitals as the fountain of pleasure. For women, they shouldn't just be the place "down there" that gives us monthly problems involving blood and cramps. Know your vagina by look and feel. Use a hand mirror to see how your genitals become aroused through touch.

While it may be difficult for those who come from cultures with strong sexual and gender inhibitions to follow this advice, do consider that cultural restrictions reflect a community at a certain time in a certain place. They are subject to change and are not the dictates of a higher power. Such restrictions are simply the means by which that higher power is being humanly interpreted.

Self-acceptance of one's sexuality can also be a culturally difficult problem for men. I have had teenage male clients who were addicted to porn and masturbation because their faith forbade them to touch their genitals. For them, it was the religious inhibition that created the problem, not their own naturally developing sexual curiosity and need for expression.

Some of my clients have so many layers of inhibition that it takes a very long time for them to break through their constraints. I have had a fifty-eight-year-old female virgin as a client and a thirty-five-year-old male virgin. It took many sessions to build up their trust before they were willing to touch themselves.

While the brain can inhibit sex with irrelevant or negative chatter, it can also function as an imaginative erogenous zone, allowing us to anticipate and heighten sexual desire through titillating fantasies. Read sexy books. Watch romantic movies and sexy videos.

———————————

Joanne was a beautiful, raven-haired woman in her late forties who wanted to rid herself of the extra twenty pounds she had gained during the past year. As someone used to turning heads, the prospect of losing her looks terrified her. Joanne had struggled through severe diets, including juice fasts, which had thrust her into a vicious cycle of bingeing and restricting. This had dredged up childhood feelings of anguish when she, as a pudgy nine-year-old, had been bullied because of her weight.

Joanne had been married for twenty years to a corporate executive. Anthony was a workaholic who spent little time at home with her and their two children. Though she had hired a private detective, with divorce in mind, she hadn't as yet found any evidence of infidelity on Anthony's part.

As the owner of her own public-relations firm, Joanne had plenty of opportunities to meet men, which had resulted in quite a few short-term flings. Joanne would lure a man into her web, they'd have a couple of champagne-and-caviar encounters and hop into bed, and then Joanne would dump the guy and move on. She described herself, quite nonchalantly, as frigid. All she enjoyed about her affairs was the seduction of her male prey, followed by her excitement in rejecting them. The more humiliating the experience was for them, the greater the payoff was for her. She especially liked it when they begged to see her again, swearing undying love and bribing her with expensive gifts.

Joanne did not know who she would be without her ability to attract men. While many women fear being sexy because other women will judge them, Joanne fanned the jealousy of other women to heighten her sense of power.

Joanne thought that she had married Anthony for love. He was handsome, dynamic, and charming, and they enjoyed many of the same things — golf, tennis, concerts, plays. She had drawn him into her web just as she had seduced other men, this time expecting the excitement to last. When she turned off because of the deadness of her sexuality, so did he. That was also when Anthony began to spend more time fuelling his career.

All Joanne wanted to discuss with me was her extra poundage, and she was especially cagey about avoiding talk of her childhood. Only after she stabilized her weight on our mutually designed action plan was she willing to "reward" me by becoming more forthright.

I focused on Joanne, age nine, when she reported having first been teased about her weight. Since she was usually well controlled, even flippant, I was surprised when she began to cry.

Both Joanne's parents had worked long hours in the family's high-end retail clothing store so that they could live in a good neighbourhood. Joanne's brother was her mother's favourite, and she was her father's. Joanne's father hired a live-in housekeeper with a daughter about the same age as Joanne. After a while, the housekeeper and her daughter began sharing meals with the family. Soon, Joanne's father was focusing more attention on the housekeeper and her daughter than on Joanne and her mother. As well as showering them with expensive gifts, he allowed them to take anything they wanted from the family's clothing store. Feeling powerless, Joanne's mother retreated with Joanne's brother into their own cozy little shell, leaving Joanne emotionally abandoned.

After Joanne's first breakdown, she began to cry at every appointment. As she told me, her brief affairs would ignite her life for a couple of weeks, then leave her empty and depressed. She readily admitted that her infidelity was payback against her husband, Anthony, for making her feel unappreciated. It was harder for her to connect her need for revenge to her father and his mistress. Though her father had died the previous year, leaving part of the family business to the housekeeper, Joanne still venerated him. She refused to believe her mother's story that he had suffered a stroke while having sex with the housekeeper, preferring to blame that revelation on her mother's early-stage Alzheimer's.

The more we talked, the easier it was for Joanne to see that her father's death had released her from his emotional grip. She also came to recognize that the re-emergence of her childhood shadow — her bingeing — had called a halt to her meaningless affairs, since her weight gain protected her from seeking another one. Here, once again, was the wisdom of the shadow!

Joanne discovered something else that surprised her. She still loved her husband. She also realized that she was responsible for driving him into the arms of his "mistress": his job.

Joanne remembered how she, as a child, used to anger her mother by pulling up the vegetables in her mother's garden to see how well they were growing. Her mother had responded, "Can't you just let them be? Feed and water them, then trust them to grow on their own. They don't need you poking around!" Joanne decided that this was good advice in regard to Anthony, and she fired the private detective. Instead of poking around in his life, she decided to feed and water their relationship.

Joanne began attending her husband's company functions, which she used to avoid, making sure she charmed the other wives rather than flirting with their husbands. She bought tickets for plays and concerts, which Anthony at first rejected on the grounds that he was too busy, but later began to attend with her.

Though Joanne's body was not yet down to her pre-bingeing weight, she came to terms with the fact that her broader, still attractive figure was partly the result of menopause. She also realized that the lynchpin of her sexual coldness was her fear of surrendering her power to tease and titillate men. She also realized that it wasn't her "frigidity" that caused her to break off a relationship, but the opposite: her own arousal. In her unconscious mind, it was better that her partner should suffer rejection than that she should enjoy herself!

Typically, when Joanne found herself responding sexually and emotionally, she would escape into her head and start cruelly judging her partner. She hated his bald spot or his paunchy midriff or his sweat. Then, all she wanted was to shower and leave. Just as with food, Joanne would restrict for a while before bingeing again.

Joanne and her husband had not had intercourse for over a year. When Joanne felt comfortable enough in her own skin to initiate sex with Anthony, she approached this seduction like any other: sexy lingerie, scented lotions, lubricating oil, a bottle of champagne on ice. That, however, was not how it happened. After an unexpectedly fun weekend at a friend's cottage, Anthony grabbed Joanne and they had sex on a couch, notable for being covered in dog hair, in the den. At first, Joanne began to think about her messy hair and her scruffy jeans, but the whole scene was so unlike what she was used to choreographing and controlling that she gave up, gave in, and had her first orgasm in decades. At least the champagne on ice was awaiting them.

After that unexpected tryst, Anthony pulled back from Joanne, leaving her wanting more of the same. It took courage for her to risk rejection by making the next advance. Always imaginative, Joanne couriered a special birthday gift to Anthony's office: a pair of silk pajama pants with a card saying that at seven that evening, she would have the other half of the pajama set waiting for him.

Joanne spent an anxious day until late afternoon, when she received back a couriered package. The contents made her cry: a honeymoon photo of the two of them, happy and windblown. Though Joanne knew Anthony kept this picture on his desk, she thought it was just for show, like so much in their lives.

When the two made love that evening, Joanne was too eager to please, and Anthony came too quickly, but Joanne loved being held, and she knew Anthony also enjoyed this intimacy. Both understood this was a beginning.

With more harmony in the bedroom, Joanne and Anthony created a secure base to deal with their other issues, including their mutual extravagance, which was partly connected to their need to create an ostentatious front to hide the bleakness inside their home.

Sexual fulfillment between two people typically makes other problems more manageable. Here are a few rules for turning good sex into great sex:

> Create a sacred space devoted to lovemaking. If this is your bedroom, then strip it of its electronic distractions — TV, computers, and phones. Permanently dim the lights. Add vases of flowers. Keep the sheets fresh and clean.

> Invent a ritual to build expectation. Light candles. "Smudge" the room with smoke from sage or sweetgrass — a Native American cleansing tradition. Take a purifying shower together to wash away the worries of the day. Prolong this with affectionate touching.

> Once in bed, stay out of the head. The moment we start wondering what time it is, or if we've set the alarm, we have disappeared from our partner's embrace, no matter

how entwined our bodies. Judgments are especially lethal pleasure-killers — of your body, of your partner's body, of your performance, of your partner's performance. Doubt of all kinds will insert a radar-proof shield between your experience and your ability to enjoy it.

Free yourself from negative parental, religious, and cultural values — including those possessed by your partner — in regard to sex.

Listen to the signals of your own body. Be real. Don't be a pleaser, a taker, or a role-player. Own and celebrate the power of your sexuality.

Use your voice. Ask for what you want. Set safe boundaries if necessary.

Look deeply into each other's eyes.

Slowly caress each other's bodies without attempting to arouse. The ears, the neck, the hollows behind the knees can be sweet erogenous zones.

Massage each other with lubricating oils.

Stay connected to your breath — it keeps you in the moment.

Harmonize your breath with your partner's.

Send a rush of focused energy to your genitals.

Give up control — surrender! A fully activated, sexually aroused woman titillates and assures her partner.

Conversely, when a man focuses on his partner's response rather than his own performance, he can hold his erection longer.

Be slow and steady. It's the journey, not the destination — the physical, emotional, and spiritual union of two people with themselves and the universe — that matters.

Let the sound out.

After orgasm, remain intimately attached. Cuddle, caress, and express your appreciation for yourself and your gratitude to your partner. Often this leads to more sex.

Always remember: Anyone who believes that sex is "just" sex has much to learn.

CHAPTER 14

SEX: FINDING THE OFF SWITCH

'm going to tell Lydia's story in detail because it brings together so many of the themes that reflect our society's attitudes toward love and sex. For every movie about long-term relationships, hundreds of others glamourize the excitement of affairs, rough sex, one-night stands, the thrill of the chase, obsessive love, and instant gratification between extraordinarily attractive people.

Similarly, gossip magazines play up the chaotic lives of celebrities — who's bedding whom, who's cheating, who's divorcing — building a star's profile as long as he or she remains beautiful and, therefore, desirable. These celebrities become our role models — people who seem to have it all yet are never satisfied, always wanting more. Proof of their power is reflected in the obsessiveness of their fans and the money they earn promoting products. Long-term commitment is rarely portrayed in the movies because, without the drama of conflict, there's no plot, and, therefore, no investors.

This isn't intended to be a rant against popular culture or how people choose to live their lives. I know from my work as a therapist that many valuable lessons can be gained from making "bad" choices. What's important is learning from the inevitable pain and suffering that follows, protecting the innocent from collateral damage, and always striving to move on, rather than looping back through the same emotional minefields.

During Lydia's first appointment, she told me that she had once had an eating disorder, but that she had "cured" it. A statuesque, twenty-eight-year-old redhead with a slim figure, she told me she was currently involved in an anguished love affair that she wanted either to push forward or to end. Despite the affair, Lydia described her marriage as a peaceful one. She and her husband, Donald, were friends, and he was a great father to their six-year-old daughter, Rebecca.

In recounting her therapeutic history, Lydia told me, "Five years ago, I had a very weird dream. I dreamt I had a vagina in the middle of my stomach. When I told my psychoanalyst, who was treating me for bingeing, he said my dream revealed that my addiction to food was a screen for my real desire — sex. I thought, 'Wow, is he ever crazy!' Sex didn't interest me, or my husband, very much at that time."

When Lydia's psychoanalyst persisted in pursuing sex as a key issue, Lydia quit treatment.

At about the same time, Lydia landed her first job at an ad agency, as a junior assistant. Her boss, David — very confident, charismatic, outgoing, and inspiring — was from a prominent, old-money family. Lydia felt an intense attraction to him, which David also seemed to feel. They began an office flirtation so powerful that during team meetings, the whole room seemed drenched with their sexual yearning.

Away from the office, Lydia spent all her time wondering what David was doing, planning the clothes she would wear to work the next day and the clever things she would say to intrigue and amuse him. Everything Lydia did was filtered through this fantasy affair. The rest of her life seemed drained of colour and purpose.

Lydia and David decided to begin their affair during a conference in Chicago. For the two weeks leading up to the conference, Lydia was so excited that she threw up everything she ate, shedding five pounds without having to starve herself. She splurged on sexy lingerie and went for a Brazilian wax. She imagined in minute detail how she and David would first embrace, how he would undress, caress, and penetrate her. For the first time, Lydia's body felt hungry for sex.

The day before the conference, David cancelled, claiming that he had too much work to take the time off. Lydia was devastated. All that kept her sane was David's promise to book a downtown hotel room for them in the next couple of weeks. But David cancelled that as well, this time for "family reasons." When Lydia phoned him at home from the hotel to plead, he was furious.

Back at the office, David told Lydia that he had had many affairs and that none of them had meant anything to him. His wife had found out about the last one and was threatening to leave with their three kids. "She'd strip me of everything — our home, our ski chalet. You can't imagine!"

When Lydia burst into tears, David callously told her, "Sorry, kid, but you came too late for the party."

Lydia's emotional nosedive forced her to take a leave of absence. Still obsessed with thoughts of David, she convinced herself that he actually wanted to be with her as much as she wanted to be with him, but that his wife was holding him hostage. She spent days reading books that would help her analyze his behaviour so that she could break the chains binding him to his wife.

Every night, she drove by his home, sometimes leaving her car to stare through his windows. She received a brutal shock when she saw that David's wife was once again pregnant.

Lydia fell into a deep depression that only bingeing could ease, and which led her to give up her job at the ad agency. Some part of her still clung to the idea that she and David were soulmates destined to be together, a mindset that made her pity herself all the more. Her bingeing became central in her life — at least gorging on sweets felt safe and familiar. Lydia gained fifty pounds, which she attempted to lose through fasting and all-day workouts at the gym. This pursuit took over her life for more than a year.

While at the gym, Lydia met Sam. Casual smiles of recognition progressed to compliments about Lydia's appearance, followed by Sam asking her out for a drink. Sam made no secret about what he really wanted: sex with Lydia.

Lydia was torn. Though she still felt tortured and vulnerable as a result of David's brutal rejection, her body yearned for the sexual experience of which it had been cheated. She was stuck in a quagmire of frustration and longing, and was needful of a different outcome. Since Lydia sensed that Sam was a man who couldn't commit, she decided that she would be "safe" with him as long as she withheld her emotions and all expectations.

It helped that Sam was so different from David and from any other man she'd ever known — stocky, muscular, and Jewish, with the sophistication that came from owning a global real-estate empire. That she was physically attracted to a man who was fifty-eight years old surprised Lydia and added to her sense of safety.

Lydia made a deal with herself: If she could sweat off ten more pounds in three weeks, she would say yes to Sam. To her amazement, she stopped bingeing overnight, then dropped an extra five pounds for good measure.

By coincidence, Sam booked them a room in the same hotel where Lydia was supposed to have met David. Though Lydia was more anxious than turned on, alcohol, marijuana, and heavy petting soon changed all that. Lydia had never before had an orgasm. Now her body felt transformed in every cell, as if coming alive for the first time. One orgasm made her crazy for another, which Sam delivered during a night of lust. Unexpectedly, she felt a deep emotional connection to him, as if they had known each other through many lifetimes.

For days, Lydia's body continued to feel a wild connection to Sam's. When he didn't phone or go to the gym for over a week, she felt as tortured as she had by David's rejection, though this was a different kind of arrow to the heart. She had thought of herself as a virgin, giving herself to Sam after only occasional and unremarkable sex with her husband. Now, as she secretly cried herself to sleep each night, hurt turned to anger: Was this silence the best Sam could offer after three months of relentlessly courting her?

Lydia was on the verge of bingeing again when Sam sexted naked pictures of himself. They arranged another hotel date, and this time Lydia had no doubt about why they were meeting and what she expected.

Over the next three years, Sam dropped in on Lydia whenever he chose, always keeping her off guard, then sexting her when he sensed she might break free of his control because of her uncertainty. No matter how many times Lydia's brain told her to say no to Sam, the rest of her body always said yes. While she'd lost out to him on an emotional level, paradoxically sex with him made her feel as if she were coming into her own sexual power. The headiness of that feeling, after years of orgasmic sterility, blinded Lydia to the severe imbalance in the relationship. When she and Sam were "on," life felt exciting and real. When she and Sam were "off," Lydia went on automatic pilot.

Sam had an erotic fantasy that he desired to turn into reality. He wished to bring other men to Lydia for sex while he watched as her "owner." By now, Lydia was so infatuated that she consented to this, surrendering her body to Sam for his complete control, and even allowing him to film these encounters. The reward for Lydia was sex with Sam afterward, when he reclaimed her as "my woman." The rougher this sex, the greater the erotic payoff was for Lydia. When Sam began choking Lydia during her orgasms, a red warning flag was raised in her head. She sensed a line was being crossed but felt powerless to extricate herself from her explosive emotions.

The turning point in their relationship came in an unexpected way. Lydia was out shopping with her six-year-old daughter, Rebecca, when Sam's silver Ferrari pulled up alongside them. After mother and daughter, wearing similar frilly summer dresses, squeezed into the front seat, he drove them to an outdoor food stand where he treated them to sundaes. What disturbed Lydia during this accidental encounter was Sam's attentiveness to Rebecca. His smiles, his compliments, his casual physical familiarity were so similar to the way he had groomed Lydia herself that she later vomited the ice cream. With her mama-bear instincts aroused, she began to fear that Sam was a man who had no boundaries. Seeing her lover and her daughter together also reminded Lydia of the risk she was taking with her marriage at a time when she had no independent means of support. These fears were exacerbated by a terrible nightmare in which she dreamt that Sam was choking Rebecca.

That nightmare brought Lydia to my office, though she didn't tell me about it during our first appointment. Instead, we discussed her dream of the vagina in her stomach, and her former psychoanalyst's interpretation that her excessive desire for food had masked a secret desire for sex. Like most of us when confronted with uncomfortable truths, Lydia still preferred denial. The closest she would come to owning the food–sex connection was to say that boredom had caused her to overeat, and that her affair with Sam had cured her boredom and her bingeing because she wanted to stay slim for him.

From my therapeutic training, I know that it's necessary to meet clients where they are with their thoughts and emotions, and not to judge them or attempt to impose behaviour. If a client tells me that she's going to leave her husband, I'm not going to make that wrong for her. If at the next appointment she tells me she's going to stay with her husband, I don't make that wrong for her either. It's a client-centred process, but with the mentoring role not to be worn lightly.

Though Lydia was not yet prepared to give up Sam, she readily admitted that he was a severely damaged human being. After doing rehab for cocaine abuse, he had transferred his addictive tendencies to marijuana, alcohol, sex, and work. As a workaholic, he had become a very wealthy man for whom no amount of money was ever enough. A sex addict and a predator, he had five children by three different partners. Three of those pregnancies, he claimed, were the result of trickery by women who wanted the financial security that came with forced commitment. When Sam wasn't blaming other people for his pain, he was blaming drugs and alcohol. While he seemed to hold the romantic idea that the perfect woman could change his life, he had established so many walls, blocks, and locks that recognizing such a person was highly unlikely.

When Lydia and I talked about her childhood, she began to see the connection between her stomach and her vagina. Sex had been the central factor in her parents' lives, which involved maintaining a youthful appearance through full-body tans, expensive creams, and plastic surgery. Every Saturday, they ran a swingers club in the family basement. During these "playdates," Lydia was confined to her playroom with a nanny, her toys, and a dazzling array of cakes, cookies, ice cream, and other sweets she was allowed to pick out for herself. Lydia resented being excluded from the mysterious excitement in the basement at the same time that she looked forward to an evening of gorging on sweet treats. Her nanny made it clear, with disdainful jibes and contemptuous innuendo, that she thoroughly disapproved of what was happening down in the basement.

As an only child, Lydia grew up both materially spoiled and emotionally neglected. The only time she felt she had her parents' full attention was when they were jealously feuding over some affair one or the other was having. Then, each of them would compete to turn Lydia into an ally, even taking her on trysts to meet their lovers.

When Lydia was old enough to understand her parents' lifestyle, she turned the full power of her adolescent disdain on them. She was glad to escape to boarding school and then to college, where she was an honours student in business administration. While her courses kept her engaged during the week, she continued her childhood habit of bingeing on weekends.

Her husband, Donald, was a business undergrad, too, with whom she frequently did projects. He was laid-back and casual, whereas Lydia was tense and focused. He was also very smart and inventive. On dates, he showered Lydia with attention without being sexually aggressive. With Donald, Lydia felt both safe and as if she were on centre stage.

Marriage upon graduation became yet another welcome escape for Lydia, this time freeing her from the anxiety of starting a career. When Rebecca was conceived during their first year, Lydia had an airtight reason for staying at home. Meanwhile, as an up-and-coming executive in the computer industry, Donald was away much of the time and seldom initiated sex unless they were on a high from partying. Though Lydia was frankly relieved by this, she blamed Donald's lack of sexual interest on the forty pounds of ugly belly fat she had gained through pregnancy and bingeing.

Lydia's parents' scathing remarks about her figure and her waste of the expensive education they had paid for motivated Lydia into seeing a psychoanalyst. That was when she had the dream about the vagina in her stomach. Though she quit psychoanalysis because she didn't want to waste time on that "Freudian garbage," she felt sufficiently motivated to diet and exercise her weight down to 140 pounds, which she could easily carry on her five-foot-ten frame. That was when Lydia landed the ad agency job as David's assistant, with its disastrous emotional consequences.

When Sam, an older Jewish man, entered Lydia's life, he was so physically and culturally different from both blond, blue-eyed David and her red-haired, boyish father that she failed to notice the critical similarities among these men: their sex addiction, their emotional unavailability, and their habit of turning their attention on and off like a spotlight. Though Lydia still felt too attached to Sam to break off their relationship, a deepening sense of her own worth gained through therapy allowed her to set boundaries with him. This included refusing to have sex with other men for his voyeuristic pleasure. She also confronted him about the sexual tension she had sensed during his brief meeting with her daughter, Rebecca. Sam confessed that, while he found children sexually arousing, he had never considered acting on this impulse. "Why would I bother when women will do anything I want?" he asked. Those cutting words caused Lydia to realize that Sam had turned her into a powerless child, and allowed her to experience what would have been happening at those swingers' playdates in the family basement. The more Lydia came to know Sam as a person rather than as another body, the more he pulled away from her. Though the knowledge that she was losing him caused her to suffer a death of a thousand cuts, Lydia could no longer make herself a lesser person to please him.

Lydia tried to use the sexual confidence she had gained with Sam, along with her knowledge of her own body and its needs, to spice up her marriage with Donald. When her attempts failed, she refused to give up sex as an important part of her being, or to depend on Sam's on-and-off attentions.

Lydia began to seek out sexual relationships with men whom she knew and liked — friends with benefits. She unselfconsciously described this new phase of her life: "I arrive at a guy's house with my little suitcase of sex toys. Maybe I'll wear my eight-inch spikes and my cowboy hat and my candy underwear, and I'll tell him, 'I'm your dream girl. I'll be your vixen, I'll be your baby doll.' I always choose someone who respects me, and I always tell him how lucky he is to catch me at this stage in my life." What turned on Lydia now was the fact that she had become the power figure in her sexual relationships.

At this point, Lydia decided to tell Donald about her affair with Sam and to let the props holding up their marriage either stand or fall. Donald's response stunned her. He confessed to being gay! Though Lydia knew this should have been obvious to her, both partners had allowed each other to wear their masks as long as they were needed. Now, feeling liberated, the couple began amicably discussing steps toward a divorce, with shared custody of Rebecca.

Lydia knew that, before this could happen, she needed a job. With the vigour provided by greater self-esteem, she landed another ad agency position, higher up the ladder than the one she had left, thanks to a glowing reference supplied by David. Lydia felt exhilarated to be using her mental strengths to creatively solve business problems as she had been trained to, rather than falling prey to her emotional weaknesses.

As I write this, Lydia has stopped playing sex kitten and hasn't seen Sam for over a year, though she still feels a powerful connection to him.

"Sometimes his physical presence is so strong that it's as if I could reach out and touch him," she says. While grateful to Sam for awakening her body, she is no longer willing to be his enabler. Occasionally, she feels the desire to binge, but she is able to turn off the impulse as she knows that ravaging her body will solve nothing. As she puts it, "I've had enough food and enough sex to feel full. I'm very content, and I don't believe I'll need to act out that way again." She is putting a lot of energy into her career and hopes someday to find a partner to whom she can commit.

Lydia's story has an ironic footnote. As a teenager, she sometimes sought relief from her shame over her parents' lifestyle and her own binge-ing through church attendance. More recently, in hopes of reawakening the spiritual side of herself, Lydia sought one-on-one guidance from an Anglican minister whose sermons she found inspiring. After she confessed to him about her sexual affairs, she was shocked when he tried to hit on her. As she told me, "Because of my history, he seemed to think I was easy and vulnerable." After confronting him with his hypocrisy, Lydia had the satisfaction of rejecting him with the same words David had once used on her: "Sorry, kid, but you came too late for the party!"

When I work with sexually addicted clients, my first task is to help them establish healthy boundaries to protect themselves against dangerous sex practices. Those who are married must also weigh the risk of long-term pain against short-term thrill should their affairs become exposed. For all dabblers, especially women, falling in love with someone who is unavailable or unsuitable can lead to years of struggling in a quagmire.

My goal with addicts of every description is to guide them to a place where they are no longer controlled by their addictions. This usually means figuring out what in their past is driving the addiction and what is missing from their present lives for which they are subsituting the addiction. Does a client lack self-worth? Does she need to be reassured of her attractiveness? Is she driven by some deep-seated sense of betrayal to seek revenge against one or all men? Is she bored because of misuse or underuse of her talents? Does she feel misunderstood, unloved, and lonely? Is this the pattern she learned from one or both parents? Is she paying her husband back for cheating? Is she merely curious? Is she secretly seeking a way out of her own marriage? My therapeutic approach to sex addiction is no different than with any other addiction. I offer a number of treatment methods. It's the client who makes the choice.

Once Lydia understood the wisdom of her stomach/vagina dream, she became hooked on dream interpretation, and she would arrive at my office each week with a handful of stories from her dreams. In one, she dreamt that she was perched on top of a weathercock that was spinning in one direction and then another. When she tried to climb down, the wind spun her so quickly she awoke in a panic.

A weathercock consists of a rooster, perched on an arrow, that a farmer attaches to a barn steeple to tell him in which direction the wind is blowing. The arrow in Lydia's spinning weathercock pointed to her wildly fluctuating relationship with Sam and her inability to free herself by climbing down, which caused her to awaken in a panic. The crudeness of the word "cock" for "rooster" spelled out Lydia's sex addiction. Since roosters typically crow with the rising sun, this dream was also a wake-up call for Lydia.

Lydia had a series of frightening dreams featuring a red wolf. Because wolves are often grey, the colour was significant. In one, the red wolf was devouring the legs and lower torso of a rag doll that Lydia recognized as one she had as a child. This brought to consciousness disturbing memories of her father touching her inappropriately when he was drunk. Her father's hair was red, which he dyed to garish effect when it began to turn grey. Lydia also remembered that she used to be frightened by the story of Little Red Riding Hood.

As a client, Lydia became very insightful about understanding her dreams. My role as her therapist was to help keep her safe and grounded. I was the barn steeple that kept her weathercock from flying off and endangering her and undermining her ability to guide and care for her daughter, Rebecca.

Many people claim they never dream. What that means is that they don't remember their dreams. If you are curious about yours, here are a few suggestions for remembering and interpreting them:

Just before you go to sleep, ask your unconscious for a dream. This may not work the first time, but after a few repetitions it usually does, because it's the last thought in your mind before you slide into unconsciousness.

Keep a pad, a pen, and a flashlight by your bed. When you awaken during the night with a dream in mind, jot down the images with enough detail to jog your memory the next morning. If you don't do this, you likely won't remember having dreamt. The flashlight will keep you from awakening yourself so completely that you can't get back to sleep. As soon as possible after you awaken, flesh out the details of the dream.

When you have time during the day, examine each image separately, and jot down everything it brings to mind. Just let the ideas flow without judgment. If an image puzzles you, use the Internet as a starting point to activate your mind about its meaning and use.

Dreams are messages from your unconscious to your conscious self.

Dreams are very personal, meaning that they are always about your thoughts, fears, and hopes.

Every character in a dream could be a facet of you, the dreamer.

We dream in visual images with meanings that are difficult to translate into words. Some we can only understand on an emotional or intuitive level.

Dreams often don't make sense to our conscious mind, meaning they jump around in time, have us do things that we can't actually do, and feature creatures that don't exist in reality, such as Lydia's red wolf. This doesn't make them nonsensical. All this signifies is that the images and characters in our dreams have greater freedom to express meaning, which is part of their value. Often a single image will have many subtle and related interpretations, as for example in Lydia's dream of the weathercock, which told her: no sense of direction, out of control, cock, wake up.

We sometimes dream "smarter" than we are. Lydia didn't even know what a weathercock was until she googled it. Such images come to us from what Carl Jung called the "collective unconscious." It isn't necessary to grasp, or believe in, the principle of the collective unconscious to make use of this information, just as it isn't necessary to know how a search engine works in order to use it as a tool.

Dreams that jolt us awake are especially important. Often they alert us to events and problems in our lives that, deep down, bother us more than we realized. What is the value of knowing this? Over time, repressed emotions lead to impulsive, repetitive, or irrational actions. They can also cause medical problems.

If something is important, we may dream it over and over in different ways until its meaning penetrates into our consciousness.

Dreams are usually triggered by real events of the previous day. Examine how ideas, thoughts, and images in your dreams reflect a very recent event or recurring problem in your life.

An important clue to interpreting a dream is its mood, and the feeling that it arouses within you. That can be the arrow pointing you in the right direction. Lydia's dream of the weathercock lasted only a few seconds, but the fact that it caused her to wake up in a panic made it significant to her. Even though the image of the weathercock held no personal meaning for her, the idea of spinning without a sense of direction is something that anyone can understand. Similarly, if you were to dream that you were at a crossroads, having trouble with the directional signals of your car, a little honest digging into your life should show you what is making you feel uncertain or out of control.

Once you begin to pay attention to your dreams, they begin to pay attention to you, meaning that they become easier to remember. In some ways, they are like a strange child who is at first shy, then eager to please. If you ignore this child, he or she may become angry and disruptive, but with the purpose of giving you an important message.

While you may find your dreams confusing, if you persist you will have breakthroughs. Always remember: You are the one who created them out of your own unconscious, meaning that you hold their key somewhere inside of you. Because they issue from a universal source, it is difficult to interpret them beyond the basics without the help of a knowledgeable therapist; however, any interpretation that is suggested to you by an expert must feel right to you as the dreamer.

At age thirty-three, Julie was a natural beauty with long brown hair and blue eyes who came to see me because of a series of failed relationships. She called herself a "passion junkie" and was always looking for a love story with a happy ending, but she found only abandonment and pain.

As a teenager in Saskatchewan, Julie had used cocaine to drown her feelings of worthlessness, and because she thought the drug would make her model-skinny by allowing her to skip meals. Starved for love, she compensated by having sex with every man who showed her affection or paid her a compliment. Though she had kicked her drug habit by the time she entered therapy, she was still addicted to the attention and affection she got from men through sex, but hated herself for being willing to pay that price. Her worry over what others thought of her consumed her every thought.

Julie described her sexual experiences with men as emotionally and physically painful because she could never fully let herself go in order to have an orgasm. At the same time, she did anything and everything a partner requested in the hopes of being loved: Anal sex? Sure. A threesome? She'd do that, too. As she described each encounter to me, she remained puzzled as to what was driving her to agree to these acts that she hated. Doing anything to please in order to feel valued was like attempting to carry water without a bucket. On any occasion when she was shown affection, she lacked the container to hold it.

It took Julie several therapy sessions before she was willing to tell me about her family background. Then, she confessed that her story was so dark and dirty she had never told it to anyone before. She also felt inhibited by the fact that she wasn't sure how she was supposed to behave while sharing it. Should she cry? Should she keep her voice emotionless and her face blank?

As a therapist, I know that the more someone represses his or her truth, the more shame and guilt become attached to it, and the more flexible I must be in order to give that person the confidence they need to fully release their anxieties. I assured Julie that there was no wrong way to feel. She should just let her emotions find their own course.

I heard the extreme shakiness of her voice as she groped for words.

One night when she was about seven, she remembered her father sneaking into her room. She remembered him touching her vagina, then climbing on top of her. Julie said that he did this several times during what he called their "secret private time." She described this as dirty and disgusting and awful, but she also confessed that her guilt came from how good it felt when her father stroked her vagina, opening it up with his finger then bringing her to climax.

Julie's story was about to take another traumatic turn. When Julie was ten, her mother woke her and her two siblings up in the middle of the night, packed them into a car, and without a word of explanation, began the long drive to Ontario. This action was not taken to protect Julie from her sexually abusive father. As Julie and her brother and sister would learn, her mother had fallen in love with another man whom she wanted to marry. Julie would never see her father or her Saskatchewan friends again. The only explanation her mother ever gave was that she was removing them from the house of a man who had never loved them, and that she was taking them to a place where they would have a better life.

Julie described the man who would become her stepfather as strange. She then added, "He was strange because he wasn't my dad, and he just came into our lives and took over as if he was our dad."

By the time Julie was twelve, she and her stepdad also had a "secret relationship." As she indignantly exclaimed through uncontrollable tears, "I was just a little girl. How could those men do that to me? How could my mom let them?"

Despite Julie's adult knowledge that none of this was her fault, this second illicit relationship greatly escalated her guilt. What was it about her that made men know they could do disgusting things to her? Though she acquiesced to everything her stepfather demanded, she no longer felt any pleasure. The frigidity that would haunt her adult life had set in.

In Julie's many failed affairs, she seemed to be unconsciously looking for the sexual gratification and false love she had found with her dad, even though she knew that, in reality, this was a taboo relationship that could never find a happy ending. The extra barrier of guilt she developed with her stepfather prevented her from ever reaching adult sexual fulfillment. With the men she chose, she continued to reinforce her childhood belief that she was worthless except to provide men with sexual release. When crying over the breakdown of each of these relationships, she would say repeatedly, "If they had loved me enough, they wouldn't have left me." To me, she sounded as if she was still grieving the loss of her father and the sense of abandonment she experienced.

Julie also frequently said, "My dad and my stepdad took my mother from me, and that makes me so angry and sad."

The fact that Julie's mother had exposed her daughter to two predators implicated her as an enabler, and suggested the possibility of abuse in her own family. Since the mother was not my client, it's impossible for me to know her story; however, it's fair to imagine that her relationship with Julie was a complex one, perhaps involving unconscious jealousy.

When I asked Julie about the reaction of members of her family to her declarations of abuse, she said that her mother, brother, and sister all accused her of lying, and that none of them would talk about it or admit that it was possible. Julie even began to wonder if she might have imagined the abuse, and if she might be losing her mind.

None of this is unusual in cases of incest. Since the wounds run deep, so does the need for denial as a survival mechanism. Even those who have experienced or witnessed the abuse may completely cut off those memories from conscious recall.

After months of therapy, Julie told me that she had fallen deeply in love with a man whom she sees as a spiritual match. Though he says he also loves her, his religion, which is different from hers, has caused him to pull away. While Julie knows they can't be together, she moves in and out of wanting that fantasy instead of facing the reality he has shown her.

She says she has taught him to stay in his heart, while he has taught her to stay grounded.

Is this impossible relationship, doomed to end in abandonment, just another means for Julie to replay her taboo relationship with her father? While the past can provide us with clues, it does not give us a blueprint. As humans, we are much too complicated for that.

Meanwhile, Julie nourishes herself by practising yoga, taking long walks, soaking in scented baths, and exploring sound therapy.

While building up her self-worth, she is demanding to know, "Who took my power away, and how can I get it back?"

From age nineteen, Nancy had been a full-time escort and prostitute for wealthy men. At twenty-four, she hoped I would help her leave this world behind. A five-foot-five brunette, she looked like a porcelain doll, thanks to hair extensions, plastic surgery, collagen fillers, fake nails, and fake everything else. She wanted to leave prostitution behind and establish a new life, because she thought she had fallen in love with a "real man."

Nancy was trained as a massage therapist, which is how her friends and relatives believed she supported herself. She had been introduced to prostitution by a pimp who at first pretended to be generous, sweet, and kind. He priced her at $150 an hour, from which he would take a $50 commission. Her job was to wait in a hotel room for the men her pimp sent her — sometimes eight in a day, which left her vagina so painfully wounded that she couldn't walk or sit. Any time Nancy complained, her pimp would beat her up.

Eventually, Nancy built up enough of a client list to get rid of the pimp. Though she was still seeing six to eight men a day, at least now she kept all of the money she made. When I asked why she would continue to abuse herself, she replied, "Where else could I make $800 a day without paying taxes?"

Once she was working on her own, Nancy became ambitious about improving her sexual technique in order to protect her sexual organs and to up her price.

With her sexual expertise down to a science, Nancy claimed that she became an entirely different sexual creature. It was as if she had an electric wire running through her, attached to a fuse that blew when overheated so that she was now able to have multiple orgasms she could sustain longer. She also practised heightening the sounds she made during her climaxes because she knew that would excite her clients.

Nancy admitted to enjoying the new sense of power this gave her. "I was able to feel like guys do when they have emotionless sex then just walk away. What I was getting off on was myself."

I was surprised by Nancy's ability to so easily separate love and sex, since that was unusual with my female clients. She replied, "It's just a job. Often, as they're having sex with me, I look up at the clock, wondering when they'll finish so I can end my work day and go see my boyfriend."

This naturally led me to ask, "How does your boyfriend feel about your returning home to him after having been with eight men?"

"He doesn't mind as long as I can separate work from pleasure. When I have sex with him, I'm emotionally attached and involved. It's totally different."

Though Nancy had clearly stated that she wanted a new life, her boyfriend, whom she insisted was "a real man," wanted her to continue to prostitute herself so that he wouldn't have to work. Though this sounded to me like just another pimping arrangement, Nancy loved him so much that she feared losing him if she became unable to support him financially.

When I asked Nancy about her childhood, she told me that her father had been killed in a car accident when she was seven, but that her mother had remarried a man who was good to both of them. The only problem was his reputation as a ladies' man. By the time Nancy was twelve, she had heard rumours about his infidelity. So had her mother, though she preferred to live in denial.

One day, when Nancy and her mom were out for lunch, they spotted her stepdad with another woman and two children at a time when he was supposed to be out of town. After a terrible confrontation, Nancy's mother discovered that the "other woman" was actually another wife, and that the two children were his by this other wife.

Nancy's mother suffered a mental breakdown, and Nancy basically lost her mother as well as her second father. She was raised by an aunt and uncle, who took her in only because they felt they had no choice.

As Nancy matured into a desirable young woman, her uncle and other men gave her a good deal of attention. While this made Nancy uncomfortable, she soon realized that she could use her looks and her body to make a lot of money.

After Nancy's attitude toward sex turned from pleasing men to having power over them, she began to respect herself more. That's when she started to talk about getting out of the sex trade, which her boyfriend opposed. During this emotional struggle, Nancy met an older married man who called her his "sugar baby" and showered her with expensive gifts. He promised he would eventually leave his wife and children in order to care for Nancy for the rest of her life. Meanwhile, he offered to pay her ten thousand dollars a month if she would be available to him, and only him, for sex whenever he wanted. He also insisted she remove all her boundaries, which included requiring that he wear a condom.

While Nancy still loved her boyfriend, the thought of never having to sell herself again was very enticing and appealing. The fact that this offer was made by an older man, after she had lost two daddies, also had an unconscious appeal to her. She decided to accept the deal on the grounds that she could get out of it at any time. She explained to her boyfriend that this arrangement was only temporary, and that they would both benefit from her sugar daddy's wealth.

Two months later, Nancy was pregnant with her wealthy client's baby. Now Nancy asked him to make good on his promise to leave his wife so that she could keep the baby and they could live happily ever after. Terrified of public exposure, the sugar daddy said he would not break up his marriage, and that he wanted nothing to do with the baby.

At age twenty-one, and after many nights of crying herself to sleep, Nancy had an abortion, then went back to her boyfriend without telling him about the pregnancy. She also re-entered the sex trade. She lived this life for another three years before entering therapy.

Despite the brave face Nancy tried to maintain, it was clear that she had little sense of self-worth beyond the feeling of achievement she had because of her success as a prostitute. Having lost all parental love and support by age twelve, she had drifted through life without a clear value system or any adult guidance. To this had been added what Nancy still experienced as the traumatic loss of an unborn child, the broken promises of an older man who lied to her, and the fake love of a boyfriend who used her.

Nancy was in emotional shock, a condition that was all the more serious because she was unaware of it. Though she clung to her relationship with her boyfriend, she didn't trust him or anyone else. All she trusted was the knowledge that she was physically beautiful, which she regarded as both her curse and her blessing. She also knew that such beauty was ephemeral, and that although still only in her twenties, she had already had too many unnecessary surgical enhancements.

Once Nancy began to put together the pieces of her own story, she started to give herself credit for having more than just physical beauty. She saw that she had been courageous in her ability as a very young person to make her way in a world that had shown itself to be hostile to her and unreliable. She made a conscious decision to disconnect from her previous life and to start afresh. This meant resuming her work as a massage therapist. It also meant leaving behind the apartment she shared with her boyfriend, and leaving him as well.

Nancy took pleasure in sparsely furnishing a studio apartment. She doesn't feel ready to date, but she has made at least one good female friend among her massage colleagues. She is also taking psychology courses to improve her therapeutic credentials. She knows that every step she takes to increase her own sense of self-worth cuts down on her need for validation from others. She also accepts what she used to see as imperfections in her physical beauty as part of her individuality as a human being.

The relationship we have with our bodies can be a reflection of the way we see our inner self, while our sexuality is often the way we play that out in the material world.

CHAPTER 15

DRUGS OF CHOICE:
AN ADDICT IS AN ADDICT

An addiction typically indicates an emotional vacuum in a person's life that yearns to be filled. Also, an addiction to one substance or behaviour is often supported by an addiction to another. Similarly, when the payoff from any addiction diminishes, the addict may make up the shortfall by adopting a stronger substance or more obsessive behaviour. Alternatively, he or she may seek a replacement addiction that seems less damaging, only to be helplessly swept up as it becomes just as bad, or worse.

Those who give up smoking often substitute fatty and sugary foods, just as those wishing to lose weight may turn to cigarettes to stave off hunger, to ease their oral tensions, and to fill themselves up. After alcohol has loosened inhibitions, it's more tempting to binge on food and unsafe sex. Marijuana enhances the sensations of food and sex. And alcohol and marijuana use may open the door to heroin, cocaine, and crack. To pay for drugs, both women and men may turn to prostitution, which then skews their views of sex. Those addicted to sex may binge on food or alcohol when they can't get their desired fix, or may attempt to curb their sex addiction by encasing themselves in fat.

All addictions take a serious toll on a person's mental, physical, psychological, and spiritual health until the underlying emotional problem is faced and resolved. When drugs are involved, it's essential to have medical as well as psychological support during withdrawal and recovery. If an addict relapses after a period of recovery, even returning to the same level of drug use as before can shock the system sufficiently to cause death. This may have been a factor in the accidental overdose deaths of both British singer Amy Winehouse and Canadian actor Cory Monteith.

Mitch came to see me because chest pains convinced him he was having heart attacks despite tests at five hospitals and walk-in clinics that found nothing medically wrong. I suspected he was experiencing panic attacks, but still Mitch always wanted to be near a hospital in case he felt another attack. That's how real and scary his chest pains felt.

Mitch, who was forty-two, married, and had two daughters, managed a car dealership — a job he described as high stress but with good pay. He had begun boozing at age thirteen — a habit that worsened as he grew older. Mitch's mother had died when he was ten, a loss that resulted in his very close attachment to his younger sister, whom he often cared for while his father worked to support the family.

At age twelve, Mitch attended a summer camp with his sister at a community centre. During free swim, Mitch saw his sister struggling in deep water. Though unable to swim, he jumped in to try to save her. Next thing Mitch remembered, he was waking up in Toronto's Sick Kids Hospital, confused about where he was and what had happened.

Sadly, Mitch's sister had drowned, a catastrophe his father refused to speak about. This denial required Mitch also to repress, repress, repress. Even Mitch's wife of fifteen years knew only that he'd lost both his sister and his mother at an early age — not the details of how they had died. Because Mitch did such a great job of hiding his feelings, no one felt the need to talk about these tragedies.

A year after Mitch's sister's death, Mitch turned to alcohol to drown his feelings. After a couple of drinks, a surge in appetite would also cause him to binge on food until he fell unconscious. The extra food turned Mitch into a fortress of fat, which placed a strain on his heart. Since he was his own boss, Mitch had so far managed to conceal his addictions and his hangovers reasonably well in his professional life; however, living in a dull alcoholic blur had final begun to affect his job and his marriage as well as his health.

When Mitch complained to me in panic that something was wrong with his heart, he wasn't mistaken. It suffered from a deep emotional gash that was bleeding into the rest of his life. Once he gave himself permission to express his feelings, he was like an auctioneer on speed. Never before had he shared his tragic loss over his sister or his mother, because his father had convinced him that men must be strong and silent. Instead, he'd staunched his wounded heart with food and drink.

After Mitch had finished talking, he pronounced himself to feel much lighter. Then he put his hand to his chest. "My heart has stopped hurting!"

As a youth, Mitch had stifled his grief to retain his father's respect — a childhood survival defence that threatened to destroy his adult life until he dismantled it. For him to seek help, he had needed a "manly" crisis like his false heart attack. Now, fortunately, he understood that expressing his feelings wasn't going to kill him, whereas repressing them just might. He committed to the therapeutic work that would drain his inner pool of pain, which allowed him to openly face both setbacks and triumphs in his struggle toward sobriety and moderate eating habits.

While lawmakers can ban the use of illicit drugs like heroin and cocaine, it's much more difficult to control the overuse, misuse, and abuse of medications prescribed to deal with recognized medical problems. This is especially the case in North America, where — according to the International Narcotics Control Board in 2010 — approximately 80 percent of the world's opioids (pain relievers) are consumed. Those most commonly abused are fentanyl, oxycodone, hydrocodone, morphine, and codeine.

In Health Canada's 2009 "Canadian Alcohol and Drug Use Monitoring Survey," about 19 percent of Canadians aged fifteen years and older admitted to using prescribed pain relievers within the preceding twelve months. In Ontario, opioid-related deaths doubled from 13.7 per million in 1991 to 27.2 per million in 2004.

Additionally, the misuse of drugs now begins at an earlier age. According to the 2008 to 2009 Youth Smoking Survey commissioned by Health Canada, 6.7 percent of Canadian youth in grades seven to twelve reported using prescription drugs in the past year to get high. As well as opioids, other drugs of choice include the stimulants Ritalin, Concerta, and Dexedrine as well the benzodiazepines (tranquillizers and sedatives) Valium, Ativan, and Xanax.

Perhaps more alarming than the misuse of medications for thrill-seeking are the individual cases in which addiction and related problems are caused by over-prescription of medications and unexpected side effects.

When Ron came to see me, he weighed 330 pounds as a result of obsessive eating, and he was addicted to benzodiazepines. Because of his morbid obesity, his GP had prescribed Xenical, a new weight-loss drug. After a short time on Xenical, Ron suffered serious liver complications. At about the same time, Xenical was pulled off the shelf as unsafe by the U.S. Food and Drug Administration, leaving Ron feeling hopeless over his inability to curb his weight.

On the advice of his doctor, Ron had gastric bypass surgery, which meant that his stomach was stapled. But when he continued to overeat to feed his emotional wounds, the staples came undone, leading to a second operation. Ron also had a vitamin deficiency, a continuously upset stomach, and nausea and diarrhea, the latter of which induced panic attacks since he never knew when he would have an embarrassing emergency.

Ron's doctor suggested benzodiazepines to help Ron deal with this anxiety. The benzodiazepines undermined Ron's attempts to curb his appetite, and at the same time, he became addicted to them. That was when Ron — at last realizing there was no magic pill or quick fix — came to see me.

When I asked Ron to share with me his early family life, he broke into tears. He told me that he had had two younger sisters, who'd both been born with a very rare disease that caused digestive problems. Managing his sisters' needs took up most of his parents' attention, leaving Ron feeling neglected. Because his sisters were extremely thin, they were encouraged to eat anything they wanted, and Ron, who was neither fat nor thin, was restricted in comparison.

In order to right this injustice, angry young Ron began sneaking his sisters' food and hiding it in his room. That marked the beginning of his binges.

One day, Ron overheard a shocking conversation from which he learned that the life expectancy of his sisters was only into their teens, if they were lucky. Ron was traumatized.

When Ron was fifteen, his thirteen-year-old sister died. When Ron was eighteen, his fifteen-year-old sister died. Then, when Ron was twenty-one, his mother died.

Ron was close to his mother, who had always encouraged him, though she was often distracted by the needs of his sisters. He did not get along with his father, who always judged Ron, especially because of his eating habits. While Ron's sisters' deaths had debilitated him, his mother's death left him feeling that a part of himself had died. At about the same time, Ron — a championship-level tennis player — hurt his shoulder. The injury forced him to give up the game. That was when he took his food addiction to another level, often eating himself into oblivion. He also started taking painkillers — for his shoulder but also to numb his feelings.

Ron's attempts at weight loss through drugs and then surgery represented a desperate effort to dig himself out of the grave in which he was burying himself ever deeper. Bingeing after stomach-stapling could easily have killed him. And then, of course, there was his addiction to benzodiazepines.

Ron's entire lifestyle needed to change. He began by connecting the dots between his childhood and his food addiction. He was no longer a kid in the kitchen, stealing his sisters' food to get back at his parents. To escape from his emotional suck hole, he had to forgive his parents for failing to understand his needs, and forgive himself for his resentment of his sisters and their short, difficult lives.

The cornerstone of Ron's forgiveness became his heartfelt gratitude for escaping the illness that killed his sisters and shortened his mother's life through worry, grief, and her sense of powerlessness. Though Ron was estranged from his father, his more sympathetic view of his childhood made him concerned that his father's health was also failing and that the two of them might not have much time left to build a relationship.

After Ron's physical problems had sidelined him from tennis, he became an avid chess player, just like his father. The two now play chess together at least once a week. Ron is also considering teaching the basics of tennis to disadvantaged youth, though he's still too self-conscious about his weight to make that commitment. The fact that he is even thinking about this is a big step forward for him.

Ron has stabilized his weight and is now working with a physiotherapist on his shoulder injury in an effort to lessen his need for painkillers. I've suggested Overeaters Anonymous as an option.

For complex emotional and physical issues, no single solution exists. It often takes a team, along with a patient's own determination, to change that individual's death wish into a desire to make his or her life count for something.

When George was growing up, his mother and father were always drunk. His mother used to get so plastered she would sometimes walk into walls. As he told me, "She always complained about everything my dad did, and since he never felt good enough, he joined her in oblivion."

George's parents endured their loveless marriage to the bitter end. As he described it, "They would scream at each other while I hid in a closet with my hands over my ears."

In our first session, George told me that he was seeking therapy because he had found the perfect wife with whom to play out exactly the same hated scenario in which he had grown up. "Once, we were in love, or thought we were. Now she criticizes everything I do, just like my mother did with Dad. We drink two bottles of wine a night except for Mondays, when I have to work late and my wife takes a swimming class."

George claimed that his wife drank far more than he did, and that if she'd stop drinking he would, too. It seemed to me that he was blaming his wife for his drinking, just as he had blamed his mother for his dad's drinking. He was counting on his wife to stop in order to stop himself.

What George hated most about his rocky, thirty-five-year marriage was its screaming fights. "It was the one thing I swore as a kid that I would never repeat, and now it's the main theme of my life. Sometimes we're so loud I'm afraid the neighbours will call the cops."

It was George's shame over the screaming that brought him to see me. Against the odds, he was hoping to rediscover the loving relationship he had once had with his wife. He was also deeply depressed over the loss of his son, the oldest of four children, who had died at age thirty-two of cystic fibrosis. Though George insisted he didn't have a problem with alcohol, he confessed that his grief had caused him to start drinking on his own to take the edge off. "I knew our son was going to pass sooner rather than later," he said, "But somehow I never expected it would actually happen."

George also confessed that visits to prostitutes were now a regular feature of his life. He had his first encounter in 1995. When I asked why, he replied, "My wife doesn't want to have sex with me much anymore. She's too concerned about her body and refuses to let me see her naked, even in the dark."

He said he had to beg her for sex. "Sometimes after we're wasted she'll give in, but she always acts like she's doing me a favour." Even then, the sex was always what he called "plain Jane." When George pleaded with his wife to spice things up a little, by trying positions other than missionary, she would say, "I'm not a whore."

I asked George how his first experience with a prostitute had been. He told me that it hadn't been life-shattering or life-changing, or even that fulfilling, but that he kept doing it because he got a big high every time he went to meet one of these women. It was exciting for him to be with someone different, even though he still loved his wife. He also enjoyed the fact that he could get away with the deception.

When I asked him how he had managed this for so many years, he said that since he was self-employed as an accountant, he could find an hour here or there to go to a massage parlour that specialized in "happy endings," or to call a service to send someone to meet him at a nearby hotel.

He also told me, "Sometimes I don't even have sex with them. I just lie beside them and talk to them, to share my feelings without being judged. Every experience is exciting, though there is always a huge *but*. I always have this expectation — some fantasy in my mind — so that when I leave, nine times out of ten, I'm disappointed. I'm left wondering why the hell I'm doing this, and if I would still be doing this if my wife and I had regular, intimate sex. I also wonder if someone exists out there who could accept me like all the prostitutes, and love me as well."

Even while George was seeing me every week, what he himself called his sex addiction took a new twist. Late at night, while his wife was sleeping, he went on Internet chat rooms and hook-up sites, like Ashley Madison and Sugar Daddy, to talk to women. During these sessions, which sometimes lasted hours, George would get off by sexting or talking to these women on the phone about sex. He was desperately seeking intimacy, hoping each new woman would turn out to be "the real thing." While this behaviour made him incredibly nervous, especially with his wife sleeping in the next room, it had become one of his biggest highs. The thrill started as soon as he thought of having a conversation, then continued while he chose the photo (sometimes fake) of a woman with whom he wanted to talk. On some sites, he could also arrange a hotel meeting for sex.

George said the women made him feel good because they told him how big his penis was and how amazing he made them feel, whereas with his wife he never measured up, which made him feel less than a man. As with any other addiction, his sense of fulfillment was short-lived, and he would end up feeling guilty, ashamed, and emotionally empty.

At every therapy session George asked me what he should do about his obsession with sex, and at every session I told him to be completely conscious and present about what he was doing, why he was doing it, and how his actions made him feel at every stage.

To me, George seemed to be a gentle, romantic, good-looking man who was in deep pain. While going outside of a marriage most often destroys it, in George's view he was taking care of his primal need and keeping his home life together. At the same time, he seemed to be unconsciously punishing his wife with his sexual addiction. Every marital story has two sides, and whatever he felt he was missing in his marriage, his wife probably felt she was missing too.

George and I talked a lot about intimacy, which, as I often explain to my clients, is a word with very deep meaning. It's derived from the Latin *intima*, meaning "inner" or "innermost." Inside each of us lies our intima, or deepest core, which allows a profound connection to ourselves and to others. It is the real "you" that only you can know, and is the most vulnerable part of the self. It holds our most profound feelings, our most enduring motivations, our embedded values, and our convictions about truth and beauty. Intimacy is not sex or even romance, and can actually be quite the opposite, since we often role-play during intercourse and courtship to try to please the other person and to live out our own fantasy.

I suggested to George on multiple occasions that he and his wife seek counselling. I also hoped that his wife would get help for her eating disorder, which sounded to me like anorexia. As I've said many times in this book, an eating disorder can shift body image in a way that undermines sexual relationships.

Though George's wife had always refused to seek therapy, George eventually came to a place in his life where his need for integrity and authenticity required him to present his wife with an ultimatum: "Either get help or I'm leaving."

His wife agreed to participate with George in ten sessions with a marriage counsellor. She also said she would think about going to a therapist for her eating disorder in an effort to save their marriage. This gave George some faith that she still cared about him, and some hope that, after thirty-five years of too much discord, he and his wife might find enough harmony to make staying together worthwhile.

CHAPTER 16

POST-ADDICTION IMAGE DISORDER: EMBRACING THE NEW YOU

The label Post-Addiction Image Disorder recognizes that treatment should not end abruptly with the giving up of an addiction. Recovery is a lifelong commitment. Time and insight are needed to help you, as a former addict, separate who you were from who you are post-addiction, and to launch you on the next phase of your liberating journey.

Addiction forever changes the way we see ourselves, the thoughts floating around in our heads, and the way we perceive reality. For those of us who have worked our way though an eating disorder, our attitude toward food doesn't all of a sudden become normal, as if our disorder never happened. Those of us who have binged or starved ourselves to near-death must learn to recognize on a daily basis what real hunger feels like, in contrast to emotional hunger or the complete denial of hunger. Though eating is now one of the joys of my life, even after many years of recovery I still must sometimes go through a thought process with certain foods or situations because of the memory of my obsessive desires and loss of control. Ice cream used to be my main binge food, but now I can walk away after one cone without wanting another. I still remember the first time this happened. I enjoyed the escape from my addiction even more than I enjoyed the ice cream. What freedom! What a miracle!

Since recovery is such a shiny goal for an addict, it's often a nasty shock to discover that the years of self-abuse may have taken a permanent physical toll. Smoking destroys lungs. Drugs play havoc with the brain's neurological balance. Cutting leaves scars. Maybe you have flaps of skin where you used to have rolls of fatty tissue. Maybe your body's struggle to survive starvation has resulted in sores that need healing, in a dry, dull complexion, or in a loss of hair.

My own years of bingeing and purging left me with digestive problems and food sensitivities that are now part of my ongoing reality. Because of these issues, I have put myself in the care of a naturopath who monitors my special needs in regard to supplements. I have found that rotating foods in and out of my meal plan every four days helps me to isolate the foods that are causing problems, as well as to avoid building up an intolerance to any of them. You may want to ask your doctor to give you a food-sensitivity test. What you find may surprise you, because so often your mischief-makers turn out to be the seemingly innocent foods that you eat daily.

Perhaps your physical appearance has undergone drastic changes thanks to your recovery, and you may ask yourself, Who is that person staring at me from the mirror? You may feel compelled to carefully examine each and every part of yourself to fully grasp your new body image. Perhaps, as a former anorexic, those extra pounds of flesh that saved your life may make you ungainly in your own eyes. What is a realistic weight for my body type, age, and height? you may wonder. Perhaps you're disappointed because, after losing fifty pounds, you still don't look like the glossy, Photoshopped images on the cover of women's magazines, or like that buff guy selling memberships at the health club. Perhaps after all your work, family, friends, and colleagues still respond to you in the same old way, even though you feel so different inside. It may take a while for them to catch up to you.

Those of you who used obesity to ward off sexual encounters may find that men (or women) are hitting on you in ways you've never experienced before. Perhaps without your belly fat, you've become a babe magnet. The body you are inhabiting is new to you and comes with a loss of familiarity, which can create an unexpected way of being out of control. This may require different ways of reacting to the world in order to prevent you from running back to the old addiction for cover. Overcoming sexual inhibition can be especially daunting since doing so involves trusting yourself enough to trust another person. This means not only making good choices but also being confident enough to risk the breakup of a promising relationship for ordinary reasons, such as that your personalities weren't the right fit or the timing was wrong. Alternatively, for those of you who believed that all your dissatisfactions would disappear along with the weight, you must learn that everything remains the same, except that you're thinner. For those of you who used sexual thrills as a reason to look forward to each new day, or who valued yourselves for your ability to attract partners, you must create for yourselves a more meaningful identity.

The reality is this: Change in the body and inner change are not always in sync, nor are your own eyes the best judge of your body image. To prove this to a client, I sometimes ask that person to lie down on a blanket on the floor, close her eyes, raise both arms, and then separate her palms to the width she imagines her hips to be. Then I ask the client to lower her arms to the floor in this same position. Every single time, when the client opens her eyes, she finds a solid six to twelve inches on either side, between her actual hips and the width she imagined them to be. The client is shocked to find how far off she is, and frankly, so am I.

Every recovered person I've ever known fears relapsing. That's your old demon-shadow hanging over you. Even as you remain true to your new goals, your nagging thoughts may prevent you from embracing the rewards you deserve.

Here is a memory-jogging list of some of the thoughts and behaviours that undermine a recovered person's hard-earned self-acceptance. It's also useful as a checklist for those who haven't yet attained recovery, and for readers who wonder how urgently they need to rescue themselves from negative thinking.

- Obsessive attention to weight scales and mirrors
- Excessive attention to photos of yourself
- Clothing that is too tight or too loose
- Form-shaping undergarments that interfere with enjoyment and mobility
- Fear of shopping for clothes

- Excessive attention to body parts as either "good" or "bad"
- Showy hairstyles, hats, and other accessories to distract from the body
- A continued interest in diets, weight-loss schemes, and body-shaping exercises
- Concern about your appearance that undermines the fun of an event
- Constant comparisons of yourself to friends or people in the media
- Dependence on other people's opinions
- Fear of other people's opinions
- Inability to accept a compliment
- Concern about body image during intimate situations
- Avoidance of sex because of body self-consciousness
- Judgments of your sexual behaviour according to other people's values
- More negative than positive thoughts about sex or appearance

Take your time going through this list, and try to remember recent situations where you may have felt upset when you unexpectedly caught a glimpse of yourself in a store mirror, or saw a photo of yourself that you considered unflattering, or fussed too much about what you were wearing, or worried about what someone *really* meant when they said they hardly recognized you. If you're in recovery, or working toward that goal, ask yourself how you would have responded to these same situations six months or a year ago. Compare your perceptions of yourself "before" as opposed to now, and imagine how you would like to feel in the future. Almost everyone — whether addicted, post-recovery, or issue-free — cares about his or her physical appearance, and it's often a fine line between this concern being a reflection of an individual's self-esteem or of his or her insecurity.

Not a day goes by in which I fail to appreciate the thrill of having escaped the shackles of my addiction. Every step I take, every bite I eat, reminds me how good it is to be me in the here and now. I'm especially happy to be free of the demands of perfectionism, which is probably the worst form of abuse we can inflict upon ourselves.

Gratitude should be the touchstone for everyone in recovery. You have come so far! You have learned so much in your reinvention of yourself! As a reminder of this progress, make a list of all the things for which you're grateful, and read it on a daily basis. Make this act about more than recovery, which is just the first step in opening yourself to the blessings of this life, this earth, this moment. Take time over each item. Allow yourself to experience the peace, love, and joy that flows from it. Make several copies of this list, and place them where you're likely to keep coming across them. Review your list and add to it.

The goal of recovery isn't just to bring you to a neutral state of non-addiction. The true goal is to clear away all the distraction, passion, and hardship of your addiction to allow you to make free choices that reflect the healthy desires, talents, and positive drives that your addiction subverted.

I've mentioned many times throughout this book our need to listen to our bodies, in regard to both food and sex. I've also suggested yoga as a body-friendly way of tuning in to the higher self. Yoga emphasizes breathing, which feeds our energy system and connects us, from moment to moment, to every part of ourselves — body, mind, and spirit — as well as to the universe. That's what the Sanskrit word *yoga* means — to join.

Even for those who don't understand Eastern forms of healing, the sense of well-being and relaxation that yogic exercises create is unmistakable. To your body, a deep breath functions like a cool glass of water does when you're hot and thirsty. Relaxed breathing also opens up your body, especially the hips, and makes you more receptive to sex. While there are many types of yoga, from gentle to vigorous, all of them stress mindfulness. Holding poses and relaxing between exercises is as important as doing the exercises. As gurus tell us, "It's the space between the spokes that makes the wheel."

Meditation is another Eastern practice that emphasizes the importance of living in the moment through concentration on the breath. The difficulty that our hard-driving, chattering Western minds have in slowing down simply proves how much we need to do this.

Western exercises like aerobics, Pilates, and weightlifting can also be a healthy part of recovery as long as we use them to strengthen rather than to beat up our bodies. Avoid exercise bingeing aimed at burning calories or losing weight. Set realistic goals and enjoy achieving them.

Recently, I switched to a gym more conveniently located to where I now live. Most of its classes are cardio-based, with the trainers pushing participants to the extreme. Though this combatant, boot-camp approach seems to please those in the class, I can see that some have already had knee or shoulder injuries, or are even recovering from recent surgeries.

During my first class, my old competitive self returned, and I pulled a back muscle while exercising too hard. I required three weeks' recovery, which confirmed what I already knew: Less can be more.

You don't have to risk injury to produce great results. Though I continue to attend a circuit weight-training class, when the trainer urges me to lift heavier weights or do more reps, I reply that I don't need to do so in order to get the benefit I desire.

Swimming, cycling, golfing, and dancing are pleasurable ways that our bodies have of paying us back for taking care of them. Sitting on a rock with our feet in rushing water, lying on the grass glorying in the beauty of a sunset, scaling a mountain, or playing in the snow with our kids or our dogs are simple, accessible ways of feeding the body and the soul. The Japanese call a walk through the woods "forest bathing."

Many post-addicts turn to the arts to express their newly emergent selves. Naomi, who was severely anorexic, opened herself to healing after she found her singing voice. She is now taking voice lessons.

As long as I was addicted, I remained incredibly narcissistic. How could I have been otherwise? All I could focus on was my body image and where I would get my next sugar fix — conflicting goals that were tearing me apart. While I might have wished I were somewhere else, I wouldn't have stayed so long in my suck hole if it hadn't been serving some need in me. That experience — the obsession, the wallowing, the struggle — pointed me toward what I wanted to do: help others to escape their suck holes. Addicts who recover often want to express their gratitude by helping others.

For me, that wish was just the beginning of another journey. I had to be willing to return to school to learn the techniques and models that would turn me into a professional. That process was very challenging for me. I'm no superwoman — I just wanted it badly enough.

Other former addicts, sensitized by their own pain, may emerge with a desire to serve others in ways already familiar. Ron, who suffered from obesity and an addiction to pharmaceuticals, finally did gain the confidence to teach the basics of tennis to disadvantaged youth. What did tennis have to do with Ron's addiction? Nothing whatsoever. You would have to look inside Ron's heart and mind to discover how the one action led to the other. Joanne, who liked to make other women jealous, is now closely mentoring a young woman, teaching her the workings of her public-relations firm so Joanne can spend more time travelling with her husband. She also feels closer to her ailing mother now that she has adopted her mother's hobby of gardening.

In order to move forward in life, you have to take the wheel and drive your own vehicle. While it's healthy to keep in touch with your therapist and mentors to prevent lapses, at some point you must stop seeing the world through your rear-view mirror and instead drive with confidence into your future. This means leaving behind the habits and perhaps even the people who distracted you. Does your current life reflect your new sense of self-love and self-respect? What do you wish to keep? To highlight? To change? If you're in a relationship, how has your partner encouraged or undermined you, and how do you intend to deal with this relationship moving forward? Has your previous comfort zone turned into a *dis*comfort zone? It's a poignant fact of life that change involves loss. The taller and stronger we grow, the harder it is to fit into our old masks and costumes.

Desire is the fuel that will propel your vehicle forward. You will also need to create a road map with clearly defined goals.

Once again, I suggest starting with a list of possibilities, and please don't leave anything out that may seem outrageous. Your goals should be detailed rather than general. Don't write that you want to be happy, find a life mate, write a book, be a fashion designer or a top executive, and live in your dream home. That's a start, but nowhere near good enough. Be specific. Write exactly what qualities you wish your life mate to possess, what type of book you'd like to write, what kind of clothes you want to design, what sort of business interests you, and where you'd like to live. Describe the house or the condo or the cabin or the farmhouse in detail. Decorate the rooms, plant the garden. And don't restrict yourself to material requests. Ask the universe for spiritual and soul-fulfilling goals that give meaning to life. Keep your wish list visible so you can see it on a daily basis. Ask the universe to give you every item on it, and be persistent enough to ask again and again. This is also a great time for affirmations. Imagine yourself whole, happy, productive, and successful in your new life.

Always remember that you deserve to be happy, and that this will happen if you have the will, the heart, and the patience to create happiness. This process isn't magic, and it doesn't happen overnight, but you are the creator of your own destiny, which is how you have worked, or will work, your way through addiction to recovery. Use all the muscles that you strengthen along the way. Know that you will reach your goals, and relish each step. Make the memory of any hard-won success a powerful tool in the joyful new life you are creating. What once seemed a big challenge will turn into a way of life.

For those of you in the early stages of recovery, as well as for those who have yet to make this commitment: Find inspiration in the stories of the courageous people whom you have met in this book. The road from addiction to recovery is a well-worn one. You are not alone, but you alone can take that first step. Change your thoughts and you change yourself. Change yourself and you change everything.

CHAPTER 17

THE IMPOSSIBLE: CLIMB THE HIGHEST MOUNTAIN

While I was seeing clients as a supervised psychotherapist intern, I would often notice Bryce Wylde, host of CP24's live TV show, *Wylde on Health,* at my gym. One day I blurted to him, "I once had an eating disorder, and I'd like to talk about it on your show."

I wasn't used to speaking publicly about my bingeing. This confession just popped out of my mouth. It wasn't something I had planned.

After a brief chat, Bryce invited me onto his show.

I was terribly nervous and excited on April 15, 2011, the day of the interview. This would be the first time I was ever on TV, and CP24 — Bryce's station — has 4.2 million viewers. Everything seemed to be going fabulously well when Bryce interrupted our interview to tell his audience about his plan to join a team that would be climbing Tanzania's Mount Kilimanjaro. The climb was, he explained, an event to raise money for Ontario's Markham-Stouffville Hospital's child and adolescent mental health services. As Africa's highest mountain, Kilimanjaro reaches 5,895 metres above sea level.

I heard myself exclaim, "I want to go, too!"

Bryce replied, "But we're leaving in fifty days. Each of us has had to raise ten thousand dollars minimum for the hospital, along with the same amount for the climb."

"I'm going," I insisted.

When I told friends and family, a typical response was, "*Sure* you are. That's crazy!"

Yes, it was crazy, but my ADHD kicked in, along with my old telemarketing skills. I phoned everybody I knew, and I was so focused and so extreme and so passionate that I raised more than ten thousand dollars in fifty days, whereas some who'd been trying for a year couldn't raise the full amount.

My GP was reluctant to sign my health certification, cautioning "It's only been six months since your accident." He was referring to my being thrown from a horse, breaking a rib, tearing the skin from my back, sustaining a concussion, and damaging my hip, neck, and spine through whiplash.

Packing for Kilimanjaro was stressful because I'd never done anything remotely like this before. Here was the list I was given: two pairs of shorts, one pair of pants, two T-shirts, one snow jacket, one rain jacket, one K-Way jacket (lightweight, waterproof, folds into its own bag), two long-sleeved lightweight tops, one long-sleeved, heavy top, one fleece jacket, one pair of lightweight long johns, one pair of heavy long johns, underwear, socks, sleeping bag, hat, mitts, and little slippers.

I added to this climbing poles, vinyl covers to protect my boots and legs from dust, a bandana, and snow pants — thank God for those snow pants! I also took snacks (the previous sixteen chapters will tell you why), baby wipes, hand and foot warmers, a lantern that never worked because of lack of oxygen, a camera and a cellphone (as did everyone else), music, makeup (more about that later), water-purifying pills and drops, electrolytes, and every imaginable pharmaceutical — I mean, I've never had a hemorrhoid in my life, but *what if* I got one on the mountain? Later, when the other climbers learned about my medical stash, I became the go-to person for every ailment.

On July 12, 2011, I stood at the foot of Mount Kilimanjaro, at 1,950 metres above sea level, with seven other women and ten men — all high-powered professionals, including six medical doctors — from the Greater Toronto Area.

I know that I often give off conflicting signals. I have a girlie side that needs nurturing, along with a hard-driven core. I'm sure most of the other climbers looked at my waist-length blond hair extensions, along with my fake nails, and thought, Who is this little chick princess? I felt proud to be my uncensored self, while planning to prove that I had what it took to rise to the challenge.

Meanwhile, the tent that I shared with a divorced dentist in her fifties became known as the Barbie tent.

On the mountain, we couldn't shower for the seven days it took to go up and the three days it took to come down. Every morning I washed my face with baby wipes, and then put on blush, mascara, and lipstick. At first, the others thought this was funny, but later they wondered where I found the energy. They also began to crave my baby wipes. I had been told by other climbers to bring lots of them, but what did "lots" mean? I had brought what I thought to be a ridiculous number, but toward the end of the climb, I had to hide them from covetous climbers if I wanted to keep clean.

Our climb began pleasantly enough, through farmlands, high grass, and thinning pine forests. We had about seventy sherpas who were always happy and cheerful, despite the sixty pounds they carried on their heads. It made my neck ache just to watch them. In addition to our luggage and our tents, they carried buckets of water and food (including breakables like eggs), and stoves and generators to cook our meals. They typically made this journey about once a month, for as little as a couple of dollars a day. Even on the higher slopes, they sang while climbing — I don't know how they managed that! They were amazing. I had such respect for them.

After four hours of trekking, our party reached our first camp at 2,600 metres. It offered sweeping views across the Kenyan plains. As energy for the climb, I had been told that I would need lots of carbs, which my body was no longer used to digesting, especially gluten. I knew I had no choice but to surrender to the situation and to assume the carbs would burn off quickly as fuel.

I often ate more than the men, even the big men. Some said they wouldn't have believed how much I could eat if they hadn't seen it with their own eyes (again, see the previous sixteen chapters). I wasn't bingeing, and I never worried about my weight. My only concern was for my well-being and survival.

At every meal, we ate soup to stay hydrated. We also had to drink four litres of water a day, purified with tablets and supplemented with electrolytes. As further insurance against illness, we squeezed the sanitizer Purell, which contains ethyl alcohol, onto our plates, cups, and cutlery, and then wiped them with napkins.

Every base camp had places to throw out garbage, and we had to hold on to ours during the climb up to each camp. We were allowed to urinate anywhere we wanted. For bowel movements, we had to use the toilets at the base camps or dig a hole like a cat does, then keep the used tissue in a zip-lock bag in our backpacks to discard at a garbage site.

Each night, our sherpas set up our tents, which we had rented from a supply company. Afterward, they would wind down by smoking marijuana and hash, which I could smell from my tent. *How could they get high each night, acclimatize to the altitude, and still work so hard every day?* That was another mystery that fascinated me.

By the second day, we could see the Kibo Peak and the ice fields rimming Reusch Crater as we headed toward the multiple summits of Mawenzi. In a single trek, we might pass through half a dozen ecosystems. We'd disappear into a cloud, where we would shiver from the condensation, then come out twenty minutes later and be ripping off our clothes because the sun was so steaming hot.

By our fourth day, we were above the level at which vegetation can grow. We camped at 4,300 metres, below the rocky cliffs of Mawenzi. During a day's stopover, we climbed along a very narrow, steep ledge to what was by far the most breathtaking scenery I've ever seen in my life. The weather was perfect — sunny and dry — as we sat at our destination, seeing the world as if from the wing of a low-flying glider. I could feel the air pass through my body as if I were completely porous. It was so still, so serene, and I felt so free that I wanted to stay this way forever. I also had moments of enlightenment in which I saw how many different paths life offered to each of us.

Our nights on the mountain were wonderful, despite the bitter cold and low oxygen levels. I remember sitting on the rocks with the full moon so close I felt like I could reach up and pull it down. The stars were unbelievably brilliant. The Milky Way was dense with light, I could see nebulas, and sometimes comets flared across the sky. I could see the curvature of the Earth as the moon slipped behind the horizon — mountains rippling on top of mountains. Meanwhile, the sun would be rising in the other half of the sky. It was mind-blowing.

As our oxygen thinned, we all began to talk more freely, as if we had no filters. People shared their hardships and their reasons for the climb, and I was very open in answering questions about my hair extensions — a fun experiment I don't need any more! — my fake nails, and my makeup. I tried to be light and amusing while keeping the more serious side of myself to myself. I remember laughing and giggling, and forgetting what story I might be trying to tell or what thing I happened to be looking for.

We often found it incredibly hard to sleep, despite the fatigue we felt from climbing. Our shared tents were only about six-and-a-half feet square and very low slung. My hips became bruised from lying on my side on the hard, damp, cold ground, and because we were usually camped on a slant, I would sometimes awaken at the bottom of the tent, squished into a ball, and with a dry, sore throat from the dust. Instead of fighting the pain, I went into it, accepting and embracing it, the way Charlene Afremow of Landmark had modelled for me.

When I did sleep, I had some of the weirdest and most vivid dreams of my life. I remember waking up feeling as if I'd resolved some big issue, with light bulbs flashing inside my head, but without knowing what it was that I was supposed to have resolved.

Many of our climbers were now suffering from altitude sickness. Someone had migraines, someone lost a tooth, someone had diarrhea. Others complained of frostbite and indigestion, hypothermia, aching backs, vomiting, and fever. A couple were like seasick geese, unable to see or walk straight. I did energy healing on them, the way I do on my clients, removing blocks and teaching them how to relax and breathe properly, hoping they'd be able to make it to the peak.

Most of us were sunburned because we had to endure double sun, both from above and reflected from below. Some people's lips were burned so badly, both inside and out, that they looked like they might fall off. I was glad I had my lipstick, which had protected mine. I didn't get sick. I was in great physical shape.

Sometimes I questioned what had compelled me to climb this mountain, but more often I felt like I was on a high. To my surprise, I loved having less. Living out of a suitcase felt so easy and so simple. All I needed to think about was my next step — not even our next destination, just my next step. My thoughts were basic: food, sleep, warmth, shelter, meditation, and bonding with the others. I had nothing to worry about, nothing to stress over. I was so free — a gift for my mind, body, and soul.

Our highest camp — on days six and seven — was at the Kibo Hut, a stone building with makeshift toilets, directly beneath the Kibo crater wall. Here was a dark, lunar landscape — very cold and with patches of snow — at 4,750 metres.

Kibo itself was shrouded in misty clouds.

While climbing, we had occasionally met other parties, but it was only at Kibo that we encountered a crowd scene. Most distressing was the toll the climb had taken on some of the sherpas escorting the various groups. One in particular had pushed himself to the extreme, probably because he was afraid of losing his income if he complained. It was terrible to witness his collapse. The doctors in our group helped bring him down to an area of safety, possibly saving his life by doing so. Since this was just before our last push, all of us were experiencing burnout because of loss of oxygen and physical fatigue. Seeing and dealing with the sherpa's suffering first-hand not only intensely aroused our compassion but also confronted us with the very real danger awaiting us the next day.

Our final climb to the Uhuru Peak was gruelling. We started out at 1:00 a.m. along a zigzag trail, like drones travelling through the dark, guided only by our headlamps. I'm sure pumping a Stairmaster at level twenty with twenty pounds of bricks on my back would have felt easier. All the black dust from the pulverized volcanic rock kicked up into our faces, seeped in our mouths, slid down our throats, and clogged our lungs. Sometimes we couldn't open our eyes, and when we choked or blew our noses, out came a continuous black stream. It was just as well that it was dark, because if I could have seen what we were travelling through, I might have turned back. No one warns you about this in the advertising brochures!

After a climb of another 1,000 metres, some of us reached the day's first rest stop at Gilman's Point. Here the landscape was even more lunar. Much of the glacial ice had melted, and we were told that the mountain would be off limits in a few years to protect it. We had another 1,200 metres to climb to our destination, the Uhuru Peak. I knew reaching it would be a test of mind over matter, but at no point did I ever entertain the idea that I would fail.

Only six of our group of eighteen reached the top — 5,895 metres! I was the first — it had taken ninety minutes. Bryce Wylde was a couple of steps behind, followed by his cousin. My tent mate, whom I'd energy healed, also made it. The other twelve at least got as far as Gilman's.

Bryce, his cousin, and I had scaled Uhuru so fast that we arrived before sunrise, meaning that it was still too dark to see the view, let alone to glory in it. We were supposed to stay only fifteen minutes because of minimal oxygen available to the brain at that elevation, but we hung around for forty-five, waiting for the sunrise. That was far too long, and it felt like hours. The lack of oxygen made it hard to talk, and it was frigid because at that altitude the cold gets into your bones. Before this climb, I'd never really known what the term "bone-chilling" meant, but now I'd been living it for seven days.

When sunlight finally struck Uhuru, I saw spectacular peaks sticking out of vast areas of clouds, glittering from all angles. I saw glaciers — enormous ones — like nothing I'd ever imagined. The world looked as if it went on forever — so vast and so cold — and the vista reminded me of how tiny we are within the universe.

For a while, I was so mesmerized that I forgot about the lack of oxygen and even the cold, because — suddenly — I realized why I had needed to climb this mountain. Less than a year ago, my father had been diagnosed with cancer. Then I had hit a child with my SUV. And then I had been thrown off a galloping horse. But now I was filled with such exaltation that I was able to blow all that physical and emotional pain out the top of my head, then send it hurtling down the mountain to oblivion.

The descent from Uhuru was anticlimactic, as expected. When the three of us reached Gilman's Point, ninety minutes below, most of our group's climbers were just arriving.

Back at Kibo, I ate a pack of figs to restore my depleted energy, then crawled into my sleeping bag in total exhaustion mixed with feelings of celebration, joy, gratitude, and satisfaction. Two hours later, I was awakened for another dozen-hour hike.

Our trek down the mountain was far harder than our climb up. I felt as if I'd given birth, and now I had to descend from the sky with my body totally depleted. I remember passing quite a few descending climbers on the way, as if we were scrambling to return to the comforts we'd left at the foot of the mountain. I was so spent that nothing mattered — not the lovely clouds, or the majestic peaks, or the endless plains.

Back home at last, what I most appreciated was running water. I turned on the tap, then watched the water flow for about twenty minutes, full of awe at its beauty. My mountaintop experience seemed so distant, so surreal.

My family and friends were right: It *had* been crazy to imagine that I could ever climb Mount Kilimanjaro. But I was also right: Sometimes in your life you have to attempt the impossible.

AFTERWORD

BY D. BLAKE WOODSIDE, M.D.

Medical Director, Program for Eating Disorders, Toronto General
Hospital, and Professor, Department of Psychiatry, University of Toronto

Eating disorders are a serious business. While the stereotype is that conditions such as anorexia nervosa and bulimia nervosa are bad habits of silly rich girls or lifestyle choices, the truth is that these are lethal medical conditions that are anything but a choice. Anorexia nervosa has the highest mortality rate of any psychiatric condition, and the mortality rate for bulimia nervosa is not inconsiderable. If you have anorexia this year, you are twelve times more likely to die than a person your age who does not have anorexia.

Beyond the issue of mortality, there is the risk of developing a chronic, treatment-resistant form of the illness that can persist for decades, robbing the individual of the chance to have a normal, fulfilling life. Such ongoing illness has devastating effects on the family and others close to the ill person, and is a terrible burden.

Timely access to effective, evidence-based care is a major problem for those affected. Discriminated against at every turn, too many people simply conclude that they cannot navigate our overly complex, fragmented mental health system and they give up trying to seek help — thus being condemned to ongoing illness.

The discrimination starts with societal attitudes toward these conditions. As mentioned above, a common view is that these conditions are lifestyle choices that don't warrant treatment or the expenditure of health care resources. Even if a sufferer can overcome this prejudice and present him- or herself for treatment, he or she is likely to come up against health care practitioners who, while well-meaning, have no training or experience in the treatment of eating disorders. Did you know that there is almost no exposure to eating disorders in medical school, and that even in psychiatric training programs the exposure is less than five hours out of a five-year residency? And that most psychiatric trainees have never worked with a person suffering from anorexia or bulimia? The situation in family practice training is even worse.

Even if the sufferer is fortunate enough to encounter a health care practitioner who is able to make an appropriate diagnosis, he or she is then faced with the daunting task of attempting to locate expert treatment. Such treatment is poorly available in Canada, with long waiting lists — even for those most severely affected. Many sufferers are forced into our parallel private mental health system, often taking out loans or even mortgaging their homes to fund treatment provided by trained health care professionals but not covered by provincial health care plans. Others are driven to seek treatment in the United States, at enormous financial cost to themselves.

Others are told that their conditions are not treatable, and that they should learn to "live with their illness." Can you imagine someone with diabetes being told the same thing? And it is so far from the truth. The majority of those who can somehow access appropriate treatment will make a very full recovery — so that no trace of the illness remains.

And a significant factor in this situation is societal discrimination against mental illness, especially in young women. Those suffering, and their families, too often struggle alone with feelings of shame, believing that their illness is not legitimate and should not be attended to. These feelings are reinforced when they discover that treatment is not adequately available.

If anorexia nervosa were an illness of middle-aged men, if it were like prostate cancer, there would be a clinic in every hospital in our country, and there would be marches in the street to protest the kind of waiting lists that face those with even the most severe forms of the illness.

Individuals courageous enough to tell their stories in public, such as the author of this book, contribute very significantly to reducing discrimination against those suffering, and the shame felt by themselves and their families. I salute this bravery as a real service to all those who suffer.

ACKNOWLEDGEMENTS

First, my thanks and appreciation to all those brave men and women who found the strength to open up and tell me their stories. Your support and contributions were both inspirational and insightful.

I am highly indebted to the people who supported, sponsored, and encouraged me to climb the highest mountain in Africa, Mount Kilimanjaro, to raise money to help build a state-of-the-art mental health facility/hospital for children and adolescents in Stouffville, Ontario.

Having written and published my first book through Dundurn Press, I would like to thank the entire crew for their support — what a spectacular bunch. In particular, I appreciate the efforts of Dundurn's publisher Kirk Howard, in taking a chance on me as a first-time author; Carrie Gleason, for walking me through the book publishing process and for her patience with helping me realize my goal; Kathryn Lane for working so closely with me and making sure *Food, Sex & You* was ready for publication; Sheila Douglas, for believing in me; Margaret Bryant, for having faith in my book and getting it on the shelves so I can share it with the world; and Karen McMullin, for seeing the endless possibility in me as an author. Above all, I am grateful to the entire team at Dundurn for turning my dream into something real and tangible.

I would especially like to express my heartfelt gratitude to Sylvia Fraser for her time, insight, and knowledge, which helped shape the message of this book. Your efforts and contributions are greatly appreciated. I also want to extend a huge thank you to Beverley Slopen for finding a home for *Food, Sex & You*.

Producing and hosting *Mind Matters* for Rogers Television provided me with the requisite knowledge and inspiration to begin writing *Food, Sex & You*. In the same light, I want to thank my supervising producer, Rick Pereira, as well as Emily Anonuevo, and the panel of expert guests who made *Mind Matters* possible. Details about the show are available at www.lovenlife.ca.

If it weren't for the incredible people around me on a day-to-day basis, life wouldn't be the same. My deepest appreciation goes out to my support team, especially my therapist M.I., who never gave up on me, even when I had given up on myself. You are my mentor and someone whom I deeply value and respect.

To my grandparents, survivors of the Holocaust, I am grateful that you have shown me strength and courage, what it means to be a survivor through and through, and that family comes first.

Dad, you always show me the way forward and are my biggest fan. You were always there to advise me every step of the way to the publication of this book.

Mom, you're my Superwoman. You have shown me true strength and unconditional love. Thank you for helping shape who I am today.

To my sisters — my wonderful, talented sisters, Jessica and Melysa — thank you for bringing colour and joy into my world. I am so blessed to have two beautiful women who love and accept me for who I am. Your love and presence provided me with needed energy and reassurance while writing. I love you two!

To my children, Tyler and Kyle: if it weren't for you, there would be far less to strive for. Thank you for lighting my fire, giving me purpose, and sharing your love.

NOTES

1. When someone has a distorted body image, they obsess over flaws in their appearance that others may not notice. Many of us do not like our nose, say, or our thighs, but sufferers of body dysmorphic disorder think about their perceived flaws continuously. Their distorted body image does not allow them to see how they really look, and they will not believe others who tell them they look fine. A distorted body image can lead to cyclical negative thoughts and emotional distress.
2. Persistent eating behaviours that negatively affect your health, emotions, and life are considered eating disorders. Most involve focusing too much on your weight, body shape, and food, leading to dangerous eating behaviours that can result in your body not receiving sufficient nutrition, and can result in heart and digestive problems and other diseases. Anoerexia nervosa, bulimia nervosa, and binge-eating disorder are the most common eating disorders.
3. Sex addicts have compulsive sexual thoughts and acts. As their sex addiction progresses, they usually have to intensify their behaviour to achieve satisfaction.
4. This book should not be seen as a substitute for medical care. If you believe you may have an eating disorder or addiction, or a neurological or mood disorder, such as ADHD or depression, seek the advice of your doctor.

5. W., Bill. *Alcoholics Anonymous: The Story of How Many Thousands of Men and Women Have Recovered from Alcoholism.* 4th ed. New York: Alcoholics Anonymous World Services, Inc., 2001.

6. Set point theory argues that the body maintains a normal weight and body fat level. Some people may have a high set point, which means that they naturally have a higher weight. Others may have a lower set point, and therefore a lower body weight. Despite dieting efforts, the body tends to return to its natural set point weight.

7. Often people with ADHD become obsessed with what they are passionate about. When that happens they become hyper-focused. For example, I became obsessed with my weight and body and so that became my preoccupation. For more information, see https://www.psychologytoday.com/blog/here-there-and-everywhere/201205/interview-dr-ari-tuckman-adult-adhd.

8. Pain-body theory was developed by Eckhart Tolle in his book *A New Earth: Awakening to Your Life's Purpose* (New York, N.Y: Dutton/Penguin Group 2005.) Essentially, it means that we unconsciously seek pain over and over again, and engage in behaviours that support our pain-body.

9. Although I saw my therapist for ninety minutes a week for many years, today I am not as dependent on her. It is the job of a therapist to help the client, but not in such a way that the client becomes too dependent on him or her. A good therapist gives clients the tools they need to make the decisions and choices that are right for them, not to make decisions for them.

10. In this context, codependency is a psychological condition in which an individual is in a dysfunctional relationship that involves living with and providing care for a drug addict or alcoholic.

ADDITIONAL RESOURCES

HELPLINES AND ONLINE RESOURCES

Canada Alcohol and Drug Rehab Programs
www.canadadrugrehab.ca

Online directory of alcohol and drug rehab programs and other addiction-related services, including eating disorder treatment centres, located in Canada.

Food Addicts in Recovery Anonymous
www.foodaddicts.org
(781) 932-6300

Outpatient recovery and support groups worldwide.

National Eating Disorders Association (NEDA)
www.nationaleatingdisorders.org
(800) 931-2237

U.S. advocacy, education, and support organization for eating disorders. Useful information on insurance issues on the website.

National Eating Disorder Information Centre (NEDIC)
www.nedic.ca
(866) 633-4220; (416) 340-4156 (Toronto)

Canadian outreach, education, and support organization for the awareness, prevention, and treatment of eating disorders.

Overeaters Anonymous
www.oa.org
(505) 891-2664

Support groups and meetings held all over the world for compulsive overeating, binge eating, and other eating disorders.

TREATMENT CENTRES

Canada

For further resources, contact your local government-run health services, or check the online directories at www.nedic.ca and www.canadadrugrehab.ca.

Addiction Canada
www.addictioncanada.ca
(866) 220-6151

Residential, inpatient, and outpatient treatment for drug addiction, as well as eating disorders and other addictions. Rehab facilities in Ontario and Alberta.

Bellwood Health Services
www.bellwood.ca
(800) 387-6198

Treatment for substance abuse, sexual addiction, problem gambling, addiction and PTSD/OSI, and eating disorders. Residential programs, detox, family services, outpatient groups, and counselling.

Canadian Centre for Addictions

www.canadiancentreforaddictions.org

(855) 499-9446

A private inpatient rehabilitation program for alcohol, substance, and drug abuse. Other services include individual and group counselling sessions, interventions, and extended aftercare. Locations in Toronto and Port Hope, Ontario.

GreeneStone Muskoka

www.greenestone.net

(877) 762-5501

Residential and collaborative treatment for individuals with substance abuse and co-occurring disorders. Bala, Ontario.

Helix Healthcare Group

www.helixhealthcaregroup.com

(416) 921-2273

Treatment of mental health, addiction, and trauma. Outpatient and counselling services. Toronto, Ontario.

Homewood Health, Inc.

www.homewoodhealth.com

(877) 798-8355 (The Homewood Clinic, outpatient services);

(866) 839-2594 (The Homewood Health Centre, inpatient services)

Homewood provides a continuum of stay-at-work, return-to-work, and treatment services for addiction and mental health issues, grounded in over 130 years of treatment expertise.

Hopewell Eating Disorders Support Centre

www.hopewell.ca

(613) 241-3428

Information, mentoring, workshops, and support groups for those affected by eating disorders. Ottawa, Ontario.

Looking Glass Foundation for Eating Disorders
www.lookingglassbc.com
(888) 980-5874; (604) 314-0548

Provides early intervention, support, recovery, and relapse prevention programs for men and women of all ages and backgrounds who suffer from eating disorders, as well as support for their loved ones. Vancouver, B.C.

Sheena's Place
www.sheenasplace.org
(416) 927-8900

Offers support to individuals affected by eating disorders, as well as their families and friends, by providing a wide range of support groups and services. Toronto, Ontario.

WaterStone Clinic
www.waterstoneclinic.com
(416) 510-9998

Individual adult and adolescent therapy as well as full- and half-day programs for the treatment of eating disorders. Toronto, Ontario.

Westwind Counselling & Eating Disorder Recovery Centre
www.westwind.mb.ca
(888) 353-3372

Residential program, online treatment, and outpatient counselling for women and girls struggling with eating disorders, body image, and related issues. Brandon, Manitoba.

United States

Caron Treatment Centers
www.caron.org
(800) 854-6023 (Pennsylvania); (800) 221-6500 (Florida)

Residential and outpatient services, treatment, and support for individuals and families affected by drug and alcohol addiction, and behavioural issues.

Residential centres in Florida and Pennsylvania. Regional Recovery Centers in Atlanta, New England, New York, Philadelphia, and Washington, D.C.

Center for Discovery

www.centerfordiscovery.com

(800) 760-3934

Residential and intensive outpatient programs for the treatment of women and teens with eating disorders, as well as teens with mental health disorders and substance abuse issues in a home-like environment. Locations across the United States.

Elements Behavioral Health

www.elementsbehavioralhealth.com

(855) 216-4804

Residential treatment of addictions, eating disorders, intimacy disorders, and mental illness. Centres across the United States.

The Meadows

www.themeadows.com

(800) 244-4949 (intake); (800) 632-3697 (other inquiries)

Wide-ranging residential programs and workshops treating drug and alcohol addiction, eating disorders, sex addiction, and trauma. Located in Arizona.

Monte Nido & Affiliates

www.montenido.com

(888) 228-1253

Residential and day treatment programs for the treatment of eating disorders and exercise addiction. Locations across the United States.

A New Journey Eating Disorder Center

www.anewjourney.net

(800) 634-1733

Partial day treatment, outpatient treatment, and transitional living for people suffering or recovering from eating disorders and co-occurring mental illnesses. Santa Monica, California.

Remuda Ranch

www.remudaranch.com

(866) 390-5100

Acute residential inpatient and partial inpatient treatment and recovery for women and girls with eating disorders. Part of the Meadows network. Located in Arizona.

The Renfrew Center

www.renfrewcenter.com

(800) 736-3739

Residential, day treatment, and intensive outpatient treatment, group therapy, individual, family, and couples therapy, nutrition therapy, and psychiatric consultation for adolescent girls and women suffering from eating disorders and related mental health problems. Centres across the United States.

Timberline Knolls

www.timberlineknolls.com

(877) 257-9612

Residential program for women and adolescent girls with eating disorders, addictions, mood disorders, and PTSD. Outside of Chicago, Illinois.

RECOMMENDED BOOKS

Anand, Margot. *The Art of Sexual Ecstasy: The Path of Sacred Sexuality for Western Lovers*. New York: Jeremy P. Tarcher, 1989.

Beattie, Melody. *Codependent No More: How to Stop Controlling Others and Start Caring for Yourself*. Center City, MN: Hazelden, 1992.

Cash, Thomas. *The Body Image Workbook: An Eight-Step Program for Learning to Like Your Looks*. Oakland, CA: New Harbinger Publications, Inc., 2008.

Costin, Carolyn. *The Eating Disorders Sourcebook: A Comprehensive Guide to the Causes, Treatments, and Prevention of Eating Disorders*. New York: McGraw Hill, 2007.

Danowski, Debbie. *Why Can't I Stop Eating: Recognizing, Understanding, and Overcoming Food Addiction*. Center City, MN: Hazelden, 2000.

Fairburn, Christopher G. *Cognitive Behavior Therapy and Eating Disorders*. New York: Guilford Press, 2008.

Sheppard, Kay. *Food Addiction: The Body Knows*. Deerfield Beach, FL: Health Communications, Inc., 1989.

Tarman, Vera, and Philip Werdell. *Food Junkies: The Truth About Food Addiction*. Toronto: Dundurn Press, 2014.

Overeaters Anonymous. *The Twelve Steps and Twelve Traditions of Overeaters Anonymous*. Rio Rancho, NM: Overeaters Anonymous, Inc., 1993.

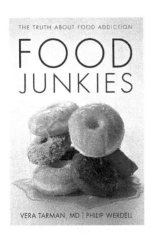

Food Junkies:
The Truth About Food Addiction
Vera Tarman and Philip Werdell

Overeating, binge eating, obesity, anorexia, and bulimia: *Food Junkies* tackles the complex, poorly understood issue of food addiction from the perspectives of a medical researcher and dozens of survivors. What exactly is food addiction? Is it possible to draw a hard line between indulging cravings for "comfort food" and engaging in substance abuse? For people struggling with food addictions, recognizing their condition — to say nothing of gaining support and advice — remains a frustrating battle.

Built around the experiences of people suffering and recovering from food addictions, *Food Junkies* offers practical information grounded in medical science, while putting a face to the problems of food addiction. It is meant to be a knowledgeable and friendly guide on the road to food serenity.

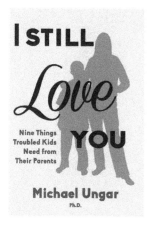

I Still Love You: Nine Things Troubled Kids Need from Their Parents
Michael Ungar

Family therapist Michael Ungar, internationally renowned for his work on child and youth resilience, takes us into his world each Wednesday, when he meets with three families with very troubled children. Here, Michael shares a side of himself that is not the all-knowing therapist: he, too, was a troubled teen, growing up in an emotionally and physically abusive home.

In the book, Michael shares nine things that all troubled kids need from their parents that will help them turn their lives around and flourish:

- Structure
- Consequences
- Parent-child connections
- Lots of peer and adult relationships
- A powerful identity
- A sense of control
- A sense of belonging, spirituality, and life purpose
- Fair and just treatment by others
- Safety and support

Hopeful in tone, and using knowledge gathered from Michael's work around the world, *I Still Love You* shows that it is never too late to help our children change and reconnect with those who will always love them.

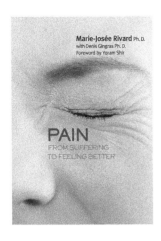

Pain: From Suffering to Feeling Better
Marie-Josée Rivard, Ph.D.

Pain strikes all of us, but it becomes a recurring or constant condition for one in five people. For millions young and old, it is a difficult, day-to-day reality, and many sufferers have been left feeling more frustrated and helpless than ever, despite medical advances.

Pain is a guide to understanding and treating all kinds of pain, and helping sufferers maintain hope for a normal life. In accessible chapters, this book explains how pain occurs at a fundamental level, both psychologically and physically, and what makes ordinary pain debilitating.

Inside, you will find:

- A guide to pain management for sufferers and those close to them
- Vital information on the types of pain, the causes, and the treatments
- Concrete advice for controlling pain, understanding treatments, and living a normal life
- Testimonials from people who have taken control of their condition

With a focus on the daily realities of suffering and recovery, *Pain* aims to inform readers about the therapeutic and psychological approaches to pain management. In addition, it offers concrete tools and strategies to help sufferers become experts on their own pain and guide their own treatment.

O 6/16
W 12/16
H 6/17

DUNDURN

VISIT US AT
Dundurn.com
@dundurnpress
Facebook.com/dundurnpress
Pinterest.com/dundurnpress